RADICAL-RELATIONAL PERSPECTIVES IN TRANSACTIONAL ANALYSIS PSYCHOTHERAPY

Radical-Relational Perspectives in Transactional Analysis Psychotherapy assesses various forms of oppression in current, historical and personal perspectives and considers the impact this has on the development and sustenance of the psyche.

Within this book, Minikin reformulates the ideas of Radical Psychiatry for the contemporary community, and honours both the historical legacy of including the social and political in transactional analysis and offers a critique of Eurocentrism in traditional relational perspectives. Through personal and clinical illustrations, Minikin encourages those in the TA community to move topics such as diversity from the margins to the centre when working with patients, and to integrate the political with traditional relational perspectives.

The consequences of becoming marginalized through alienation speaks across multiple disciplines in social sciences, making this a must-read for counsellors, psychotherapists and other applied psychologists who want to think more deeply about social responsibility within their work.

Karen Shireen Minikin is a Transactional Analysis psychotherapist and supervisor in private practice in West Somerset, UK. She is a Course Director for Psychotherapy at the Iron Mill College in Exeter She is also a co-editor for the Transactional Analysis Journal and the journal, Psychotherapy and Politics International.

INNOVATIONS IN TRANSACTIONAL ANALYSIS

Theory and Practice

Series Editor: William F. Cornell

This book series is founded on the principle of the importance of open discussion, debate, critique, experimentation, and the integration of other models in fostering innovation in all the arenas of transactional analytic theory and practice: psychotherapy, counseling, education, organizational development, health care, and coaching. It will be a home for the work of established authors and new voices.

https://www.routledge.com/Innovations-in-Transactional-Analysis-Theory-and-Practice/book-series/INNTA

RADICAL-RELATIONAL PERSPECTIVES IN TRANSACTIONAL ANALYSIS PSYCHOTHERAPY

Oppression, Alienation, Reclamation

Karen Shireen Minikin

Routledge
Taylor & Francis Group

LONDON AND NEW YORK

Designed cover image: Leigh Cripps, 2017

First published 2024
by Routledge
4 Park Square, Milton Park, Abingdon, Oxon OX14 4RN

and by Routledge
605 Third Avenue, New York, NY 10158

*Routledge is an imprint of the Taylor & Francis Group, an informa
business*

© 2024 Karen Shireen Minikin

British Library Cataloguing-in-Publication Data
A catalogue record for this book is available from the British Library

Library of Congress Cataloguing-in-Publication Data
Names: Minikin, Karen, author.
Title: Radical relational transactional analysis / Karen Minikin.
Description: Abingdon, Oxon ; New York, NY : Routledge, 2024. |
Series: Innovations in transactional analysis | Includes bibliographical
references and index. |
Identifiers: LCCN 2023014441 (print) | LCCN 2023014442 (ebook) |
ISBN 9780367256975 (hardback) | ISBN 9780367256982 (paperback) |
ISBN 9780429289231 (ebook)
Subjects: LCSH: Transactional analysis. | Alienation (Social
psychology) | Social psychiatry. | Psychotherapist and patient.
Classification: LCC RC489.T7 M564 2024 (print) | LCC RC489.T7
(ebook) | DDC 616.89/145--dc23/eng/20230627
LC record available at https://lccn.loc.gov/2023014441
LC ebook record available at https://lccn.loc.gov/2023014442

ISBN: 978-0-367-25697-5 (hbk)
ISBN: 978-0-367-25698-2 (pbk)
ISBN: 978-0-429-28923-1 (ebk)

DOI: 10.4324/9780429289231

Typeset in Times New Roman
by MPS Limited, Dehradun

CONTENTS

CONTENTS

ACKNOWLEDGEMENTS

I wish to acknowledge significant people that have supported me backstage in developing my mind and finding the confidence to express myself. I honour the trainers who have taught me and my previous supervisors and therapists. I thank Suzanne Boyd for her ongoing care and support. Deep gratitude to Carole Shadbolt, Victoria Baskerville, and Helen Rowland for being political allies. Special fond thanks to my friends and colleagues Keith Chinnock, Briony Nicholls, Marion Umney, and Paula Dishman. The love, wisdom, and support of the BAATN Leadership group has been and continues to be a precious resource: Eugene Ellis, Jayakara Beverley Ellis, Carmen Joanne Ablack, Rotimi Akinsete, Poppy Banerjee, Dennis Carney, Mickey Peake, Robert Sookhan, and Ian Thompson. Also, our retired BAATN leader, Isha McKenzie-Mavinga and our departed, still beloved Arike, aka Stan Grant.

I am most grateful to the editor of this series, Bill Cornell for his patience, insight, and wonderful mind. My mentors laid significant foundations for my capacity to think, speak, and write—Suhith Shivanath, Keith Tudor, and Richard Morgan Jones. My stepfather Victor Minikin showed me how to hold the power of your convictions. My mother Ena Elkington Minikin delivered strength and courage during difficult times. I appreciate my father, Arif Hussain, who has an exceptional mind, survived the West, and has modelled good grace in old age. Finally, and most importantly, I thank my husband, Nicholas Cole for his ongoing tolerance of my irritating habits and his support and love for twenty-five years.

Karen Shireen Minikin

Part I

ALIENATION

1

WHY RELATIONAL? WHY RADICAL?

I came into training as a counsellor having had some help with a relationship breakdown that I was struggling to understand and come to terms with. Finding it helpful, I felt hungry to better understand my closest relationships. I never did intend to become a professional, but having found the training enlightening, the placement work satisfying, I felt compelled to learn more and I continued to train as a psychotherapist. Looking back to that personal relationship, nearly 30 years ago, that experience and the subsequent separation had enacted a level of relational trauma and loss that I simply couldn't find words for. Drawing from Transactional Analysis (TA), we might think that it had reached my script protocol[1]. It had captured the deepest transferences I might have been left with following early infant relationships with my parents and possibly it touched something beyond that too. The loss affected me profoundly, physically and emotionally; it was a psychic breakdown. In terms of practicalities, a year of counselling helped me return to work and build some resources, and four years of Transactional Analysis psychotherapy helped me to restore some self-confidence and start a new relationship. Fifteen years of group and individual analysis helped me connect with the meaning of the loss and a capacity to feel more at home in my body. These therapies have been of lifelong importance, and I have needed them alongside a growing feeling of connectedness and concern about the wider world.

Having described the personal draw to enter the world of psychotherapy, I move on now to account for my interest in social, historical, and political contexts. I explain how and why I was drawn to exploring these domains in my work as a psychotherapist. Finally, I write about the connections these have within my field of psychotherapy: Transactional Analysis.

Social and Political Context

From early adolescence, I have been socially and politically engaged. In clinical practice, I have felt the pull to account for the contextual social history of clients and their family members. Whilst psychotherapy pays attention to how social and relational events have influenced the mind, there

DOI: 10.4324/9780429289231-2

3

has tended to be a greater focus on the mother/infant dyad with less attention paid to the context, the holding environment, and the normative narratives that hold our mothers and the socio-political climate that we are born into. When Keith Tudor introduced me to the ideas from Radical Psychiatry in 2002, the alienation formula spoke to me in a profound way. The original training I undertook did not treat alienation as a central focus in clinical work. However, I continued to go back and forth with the ideas, as a student and after receiving my qualification. Radical psychiatry and the ideas therein were a link back to my political involvement as a teenager in the 1970s and unbeknown to me at the time, were also a link to my father. Alongside my emerging interest in radical psychiatry, I continued in personal analytical psychotherapy and took on professional roles in the TA community. These roles and my personal work were challenging and helped me learn and develop as a woman and as a practitioner. The political choices made in the UK and the USA since 2015 have also affected me, highlighting my commitment to anti-oppressive stands and my compulsion (at times) to examine power dynamics. For those unfamiliar with this theory, the alienation formula is a way of describing the key social and psychological difficulties that people have. Steiner et al. (1975, p. 12) honoured Hogie Wyckoff for her work with this formula:

Oppression + Deception = Alienation

The idea that alienation is at the root of all social and psychological distress is a profound and simple idea that I test out frequently. I have yet to experience a case where the premise cannot be applied. With clients, alienation can offer an anchor for how I contemplate our struggles. Oppression can speak to the scripting process which is often an adaptation to the power base in families and societies. Deception describes the confusion that has been set up in our minds, as we relinquish emotional states and the behaviours accompanying them to maintain key relationships. As we need to survive within a social system, we forego some of our sensitivities, integrity, and, at times, dignity in the world we occupy. Deception and oppression are useful ways of thinking about scripting, object relations, and intersubjective processes between people as well as our wider systemic dynamics.

When Steiner et al. were developing their ideas about alienation, they summarised that alienation was a culmination of two processes: "oppression" + "deception". To my mind, this is a relational experience and the assertion that alienation is at the core of all social and psychological distress is a radical statement. It is radical because to accept it means we have to pursue a journey of deconstructing our premise and therefore our approach in social and psychological disciplines. It is relational in that it signifies a relationship, an encounter, and a subjective response. The alienation formula means that there needs to be an oppressor and an oppressed, a "doer and a done to" (Benjamin, 1988, p. 2017). Transactional Analysis has taken on some of this dynamic in the analysis of the scripting process. Traditionally, the Child has been seen as the victim to the persecution or neglect of the parents, which formulates in a series of oppressive adaptations such as drivers[2], injunctions[3], and script decisions. What has often been missing in this analysis is any reference to the socio-economic and political context of the family. However, classical Transactional Analysis did implicitly understand that there is a more powerful person with a more vulnerable one and this creates opportunity for oppression in the scripting process. This interpersonal reality has parallels with the wider global perspective and that is why I will move between history, context, and personal dynamics in this book. Having explained how the significance of radical and relational has applied to me personally, I now turn to the paradigm for the psychotherapy I do: Transactional Analysis. The history and the philosophy of this body of theory is also relevant and what follows adds to how and why a radical relational approach matters to me.

Claude Steiner and the Early Days of Transactional Analysis

Claude Steiner studied and worked with Eric Berne. He was part of a key professional group that helped Berne formulate his new theory of 'Transactional Analysis', initially for psychotherapy from the 1950s and through the 1960s. These must have been exciting and creative times for this team as a new body of theory evolved. I imagine those that were involved with the regular Tuesday night social psychiatry seminars developed strong personal and professional bonds. Perhaps there was something of the feelings and moods of this group that founded the sort of culture that has evolved in the Transactional Analysis community. It has always been an interpersonal theory taught and executed with an emphasis on meaningful relations that have created professional and personal bonds. In the last decade of his life, Steiner (2008) wrote:

> What is it about Berne's transactional analysis that so attracts people? Is it the simplicity of its concepts? His rebelliousness? The zany, provocative nature of Eric's language? The second- and third-generation writings of Harris, James, Steiner, Dusay, Karpman, English, the Gouldings, and Stewart and Joines? Is it the enthusiasm and methods of its many teachers or the missionary zeal of its trainers? Is it the elaborations of relational, psychoanalytic, and integrative transactional analysis? Is it the opportunity it offers to become a therapist and make a living? Or is it the friendly, cooperative, open-minded attitude of the people in the movement?
>
> (p. 214)

Transactional Analysis was formed in the United States after Berne, following 15 years of training, was refused admission to the San Francisco Psychoanalytical Institute. The rejection seemed to inspire a rebellious, though productive response. Since then, Transactional Analysis has developed into a body of writing that offers clarity concerning the complexity of human relations and answers about how to alleviate social and psychological pain. As Steiner (2008) stated, it has at times attracted 'missionary zeal' amongst trainers. So, it has grown, spread, and enjoyed much success since its formation in California. There are now Transactional Analysis establishments and practitioners across four professional fields (counselling, psychotherapy, educational, and organisational) in all continents. Given this diversity, the range of how Transactional Analysis is thought about, used, and developed has grown. However, what is common to all Transactional Analysis trainings is a subscribing to the three philosophical premises that were established and continue on decades afterwards. These warrant some review given that we are more than 70 years on. So, I consider both the virtues and difficulties that I have witnessed and encountered. I take a political and radical lens considering both overt and covert power dynamics at structural and interpersonal levels.

Eric Berne was seen as a maverick by his psychoanalytical colleagues. He was radical in his methodology, inclined to humanistic values, and possibly had socialist sympathies. If he did, expression of such views may have been quashed during President Eisenhower's reign when the fear of socialism was at one of its heights. Berne was somebody who evoked and provoked systemic change. In particular, his way of working, such as his open communication and contracting (Berne, 1972), challenged the balance of power in medical institutions and was an expression of egalitarianism and respect for the humanity of people. For me, personally, Berne has been an enigmatic character, hard to get to know—hearing about him through the eyes of others, as well as his writing. He was a man who, like the rest of us, embodied his history, culture, and era. I am part of his legacy—a fourth generation Transactional Analyst. I endeavour to continue his radical beginnings.

From these roots, Transactional Analysis has developed a diverse body of theories with breadth and depth of its four applications in terms of theory and methodology. The goal of all these applications is autonomy; comprising of awareness, spontaneity, and capacity for intimacy (Berne, 1964). It is important to briefly explain that autonomy alone is a Western concept privileging the experience and agency of the individual and minimising the significance of the group, society, and the context. By clarifying what Berne meant by autonomy, that is awareness, spontaneity, and capacity for intimacy, (Berne, 1964, pp. 158–161) we see his support for consciousness generally and a valuing of expression and satisfying interpersonal relationships. Underpinning this goal of autonomy are the philosophical premises of Transactional Analysis.

Three Philosophical Premises

Everyone who has encountered Transactional Analysis in a formal capacity will know the three philosophical principles: "I'm OK/you're OK", people can think, and people can change. Traditionally, Transactional Analysis theory, like the era it was born into, was upbeat and optimistic. With a goal of autonomy and a belief in treating each other with mutual respect, we have worked hard to taboo games (see Berne, 1964; or 'acting out' defensively—my definition) and enactments (eruptions of a traumatic nature; see Novak, 2015). In Jungian psychology, our efforts to behave well could be interpreted as a defence against the shadow. This may be changing in some forms of contemporary Transactional Analysis which has sought a different inquiry into psychological states. Many integrative, co-creative, and relational practitioners (see Cornell & Bonds-White, 2001; Erskine, 1993; Hargaden & Sills, 2002; Little, 2013; Summers & Tudor, 2000, 2015) have been interested in the need to make space for symbolic and nonverbal communications—even if they seem primitive and unformulated (Stern, 2011). Some developments in the professional and academic canon have struggled to permeate the culture in the international Transactional Analysis community. This means developments within the wider international community have developed but have not always linked up and been debated fully enough so that at least there could be understanding even if disagreement continued. I imagine this is true of all professions and all communities; that we struggle with competition, rivalry, and conflict, becoming more invested in our own positions than in striving to understand the other. In this light, as a parallel to our current social and political global climate, I take the opportunity to review the three philosophical premises in Transactional Analysis which are meant to drive what we do and how we do it.

"I'm OK/You're OK": Macro and micro perspectives

"I'm OK/You're OK" is a simple and catchy statement that became the title of a best-selling self-help book (Harris, 1967) shortly after Berne's death. This first premise has been a champion in Transactional Analysis and probably the most quoted inside and outside of our community. The sense and spirit of this premise is to promote holding respect for ourselves and respect for the other. The message speaks to the interpersonal roots of Transactional Analysis and its promotion of 'healthy' Adult functioning. By this, it is meant the achievement of autonomy has been acquired and that people are relating from one Adult ego state to another, which places enormous pressure on people to be conscious of themselves. This seems important; yet, I place 'healthy' in quotation marks because I think, above all, this is the premise that people feel most pulled to adapt to. In other words, "I'm OK/You're OK" has at times been used as dogma, losing the depth of its intention, and igniting politeness in our community rather than genuine congruent relatedness.

It is possible that the conflict with the psychoanalytical body that evoked the formation of Transactional Analysis has rumbled on through the decades. "I'm OK/You're OK" is always difficult when we feel our core values and beliefs are being challenged. Whilst Berne and English came from psychoanalytical roots, some of their contemporaries (i.e., Claude Steiner, Steve Karpman, and John [Jack] Dusay) leaned towards a quest for emotional literacy and respectful behaviour. Over the years, these and other writers encouraged Transactional Analysis to take more of a cognitive behavioural direction—a direction that has since been challenged by new and, at times, conflicting perspectives.

As with many theories that start with creative thinking and a capacity to push and extend the boundaries of thought, they become introjects in the minds of students and subsequent generations of practitioners. In my era, I have seen some honourable striving for understanding, empathy, and collaboration at times of difficulty and conflict. With that has come an orientation to seek to understand the other and heal ruptures. I have also witnessed as student, teacher, and participator in our community, an adaptation to this introjected, yet not quite metabolised premise. This, to my mind, has been an expression of racket feelings (English, 1971) and behaviours (Erskine & Zalcman, 1979), or the false self as described by Winnicott (1960); my interpretation being that anxiety and aggression are covered over by expressions of warmth and friendship. As with many modalities, a professional community has developed in Transactional Analysis. We have our regional, national, and international cultures. These are all relationally bound with a generic norm that has developed from our philosophical principles. "I'm OK/You're OK" becomes problematic at times of conflict, envy, rivalry, and competition. These feelings are different from straightforward anger that is more accessible to our conscious minds. In relations within our communities, nationally and internationally, I have witnessed an evasion of aggression and a desire to heal sometimes before the root of the problem has really been grasped. This has led to temporary relief of anxiety whilst toxic processes stay underground rumbling away till the next time. In these scenarios, I propose that "I'm OK/You're OK" becomes a rule rather than a premise that is genuinely strived for. Hence, the simple, straightforward language in Transactional Analysis can be misleading at times. In other words, to experience this premise at depth makes demands on people to process, labour, and honour self-interest whilst searching and pushing ourselves to understand the other (or 'those others'). A philosophical premise that becomes a 'rule' runs the risk of becoming an oppressive misuse of a good idea.

Transactional Analysis is grounded in the interpersonal, yet Berne used his ideas in radical ways to challenge the medical institution. Other Transactional Analysts have also turned to social psychiatry roots to bring

8

in the relevance of context, society, and politics. Hence, accounting for 'we-ness' as well as the 'I' has been an important component in Transactional Analysis and Berne's extension to "we're OK/they're OK (or not OK)" has been picked up extensively by Tudor (2016).

To emphasise the complexity and depth of I am OK/you're Ok, we can consider the protests that took place around the world after the death of George Floyd. Whilst well-meaning people may agree this is a death that should not have happened ('I' psychology), his death is an example of transgenerational trauma and the persistence of the hate that accompanies 'othering'. The protests and various responses to them speak to how challenging it is to live collectively by egalitarian principles because we are in a world that is not equal. For those with privilege in societies, all the time systematic oppression is sustained and functioning, there can be little incentive to labour with their minds long enough or hard enough to metabolise the collective traumas that continue through the generations. This is perhaps a reflection that those with more power in society are the groups that get to define 'OK-ness'—which then is bestowed upon or withheld from certain groups or behaviours. This is a socio-political perspective about power dynamics which has some differences to our liberal humanistic philosophy. Hence, "I'm OK/You're OK/They're OK" is honourable, simple, and potentially meaningful as an ideological premise. It is one that most well-meaning people would agree to. Living it in a congruent and meaningful way is a deep-set challenge—personally, socially, politically, and internationally.

People can think

The premise that people can think came about in part from Berne's commitment to promoting the health of psychiatric patients. He understood his patients as adults who had their own minds but were afflicted by the ways in which they felt compelled to cope in the world. Writing people off with a psychiatric diagnosis and committing them to a lifetime of medication was something that Berne opposed, and he used radical practice to challenge the hospital where he worked. Whilst this premise has been used to promote the resources and sanity in people, it is also the premise that, currently, most interests me.

Claude Steiner picked up on this premise and explored it more deeply when he started a personal and professional relationship with Hogie Wyckoff, an economics and politics student. Together with others, they formulated their thinking about the systemic influence of capitalism and the impact that has on the minds of the people. They named and developed their thinking about the psychological condition of alienation, as described by Karl Marx (1967).

> Extended individual psychotherapy is an elitist outmoded as well as nonproductive form of psychiatric help. It concentrates the talents of a few on a few. It silently colludes with the notion that people's difficulties have their source in them while implying that everything is well with the world ... People's troubles have their source not within them but in their alienated relationships, in their exploitation, in polluted environments, in war, and in the profit motive.
>
> (Steiner et al., 1975, pp. 3–4)

Steiner et al.'s (1975) definition of alienation comprised both oppression and deception. Oppression minimised a sense of autonomy of the other. They understood this misuse of power as systemically coercing people into adapting to the power base, whether that be an individual, group, institution, or society at large.

The significant contribution they made to the idea of the oppressed people was that they were not meant to realise they were oppressed. In other words, their capacity for thinking was impaired by the deception that accompanied the oppression. So, people were lied to about their internal experience, and lied to about external events such as the rationale for particular decisions, the nature of people in society, and political/cultural systems that people were dependent on. I expand on the point about deception in Chapter Four. Suffice to say that the alienation formula is intended to expand consciousness. It is an ally of deconstruction and enquiry into normative structures and processes. Hence, as the book continues, I draw in examples of how this has emerged in personal, social, and therapeutic encounters.

Simple though it may be, the most important philosophical premise for me is that *people can think*. Without thinking, people cannot change or respect otherness. The notion that people can think equips me to push myself to think and to help others think. Developing minds that can stretch, reach, and expand offers potential hope. In its broadest and deepest sense, it serves the purpose for me, as philosophically I can believe that this is what I am commissioned to do in my work. The effort it takes to claim at least some of our own minds so that we can feel, experience, question, learn, be curious, and, where needed, have meaningful thought-provoking discussions that may help us solve complex problems. As a relational psychotherapist, I do what I can to help people metabolise, mentalise, and relate. Without this ability, people cannot think well as fear, hatred, and unprocessed loss floods our psychic systems. Writing as a relational, social, and political psychotherapist, it is our capacity to think in the fullest sense that offers me hope.

People can change

People can change is a direct message of optimism; one that is reflected in Transactional Analysis as a body of theory with much investment in hope.

We need to hang on to the light of change in times of despair, as in the words of inspiration and encouragement by Martin Luther King: "Darkness cannot drive out darkness; only light can do that. Hate cannot drive out hate; only love can do that." (Luther King Jr., 1963, p. 37).

This may feel hard to do at times. At the time of composing these premises, Transactional Analysis was situated in the liberal state of California, the civil rights movement was happening, and there was a movement of growing international liberalism. It was into this era that I was born and perhaps that says something of my personal draw to political forms of liberation.

Much as I am the same as the politically engaged teenager marching against racism in the United Kingdom in the 1970s, I am also changed. I waver and swing much more between hope and despair. I see the magnitude of our systemic organisation of economic and global power, and recognise that as individuals we cannot challenge the scale and complexity of this without collective action. Even if a collective uprising was possible, I struggle to believe that there will be enough restructuring and change for a greener, safer, kinder, and more egalitarian world. It seems to me that the people and institutions that hold power do their best to hang on to it and it takes one mighty revolution, like the civil rights movement, to effect meaningful change. The process of change can be slow, the process of recovery from trauma long and arduous—nonetheless, we cannot 'not' believe. From our consultation rooms to the streets, we see people expand and flex their minds, we see the processes of oppression and deception being challenged. It can only happen through relationships, collaboration, and, at times, mutual pain. As a psychotherapist, if I believe in recovery, I have to believe that psychological change is possible. It is probably true I feel more confident in this in my consulting room than I do as a citizen. As a citizen, I feel more in touch with the magnitude of systemic power, the sustenance and dependency on capitalism, and the repetition of traumatic dynamics as I watch the news items on the death of George Floyd and the ensuing fury that has erupted. My learning, as a psychotherapist, is that psychological change needs a context and mental health is a systemic issue.

Transactional Analysis Today

We will not create change without getting our hands dirty, our pride bruised, our frames of reference shaken.

(Cornell, 2018, p. 109)

Earlier in this chapter I referred to the eclectic nature of Transactional Analysis. The simplicity of our terms and language was in part a rebellion against the use of enigmatic language and elitism within psychoanalytical quarters. I almost hear the cry from my professional ancestors, 'let the people understand!' The capacity our pioneers had to portray complexity in a simple and clear manner has been invaluable socially, institutionally, and clinically. It meant people from all walks of life can be attracted to Transactional Analysis and can use it to help their understanding of their minds and their relationships. This legacy has also been a source of frustration. It has facilitated a myth that Transactional Analysis is superficial, is all about 'Parent, Adult, and Child' and "I'm OK/You're OK". In the United Kingdom health care system (the National Health Service), it is not a recognisable treatment for mental health. Amongst other professionals, who have caught aspects of the ideas, it can sometimes be seen as oversimplistic and cognitive. Thus, the original scripting process that led Berne to leave the analytical community, feeling unappreciated and misunderstood, continues.

Since Berne's day, Transactional Analysis has expanded the core models to keep it relevant with the times, with scientific developments as well as developments in the clinical field. Drawing from psychoanalysis, there is an emphasis on the goal of awareness and insight through reaching the unconscious via transference and dreams (see, e.g., Blackstone, 1993; Bowater, 2003; Moiso, 1985; Novellino, 2005). There has been an integrative movement interested in self-psychology and the importance of empathy and attunement. The range of writers within an integrative tradition include Barbara Clark (1991), Petruska Clarkson (1993), and Richard Erskine (1993). There has been the innovative launch of co-creative Transactional Analysis (Summers & Tudor, 2000, 2015), drawing on mutual conscious and unconscious influence and bringing together psychodynamic, political, and person-centred perspectives in Transactional Analysis. Contemporary Transactional Analysis is also influenced by the relational movement in psychoanalysis and, with this, has been compelled by a depth in understanding subjective and unconscious relating, with a focus on transference and countertransference (see, e.g., Hargaden & Sills, 2002).

There is another movement emerging within our field—that of context. Back to socio-political roots, Transactional Analysis is finding ways to think and write about the concerns of our time and the psychological and social responses (e.g., Cornell, 2018; Minikin, 2018; Sedgwick, 2021). In terms of my identity as a Transactional Analyst, I have learnt in the tradition of relational psychotherapy and developed a political and psychodynamic leaning as psychotherapist, supervisor, and trainer. This growth has been an important development for me in metabolising and accounting for a personal history and legacy that takes on new meanings and purpose.

Conclusion

Transactional Analysis is an integrative therapy that has needed to open its doors to other modalities, contribute to them, and mostly learn from them. It has been available to learn from both humanistic and psychoanalytical camps. It has been at risk of being eclectic and so has experienced an ongoing struggle with identity. The three philosophical premises are potentially meaningful and important. However, in leaning towards clarity and universality, we have risked becoming superficial. For these premises to stand up to the spirit in which they were formulated, they need to be thought and talked about with the complexity and depth to which this body of theory was born.

I turn now to the core idea in radical thinking. That is the premise that alienation is at the root of all social and psychological distress[4].

Notes

1 This refers to the earliest experiences of bonding, attachment, and separation thought to be laid down in the young pre-verbal infant. In Transactional Analysis, we consider that protocol lays the foundation for script. Script refers to defences that are unconsciously created and from which the individual develops their narrative that helps navigate family, society, and life experiences.
2 Drivers of social adaptations are the tactics we use to be acceptable to others. In many TA texts they are said to form during the verbal stage of development. Personally, I think they can operate in a more primitive way given that pleasing important people in the family is a feature for all mammals that live in groups.
3 Injunctions are the prohibitive nonverbal messages communicated from authority figures in social contexts and key caretakers in families. These communicate the conditions required for survival and indicate the limitations of the parents. The injunction "Don't Exist" is considered the most serious and would indicate a caretaking environment that was dangerous and/or neglectful in terms of basic needs.
4 A version of this chapter was published in *Psychotherapy and Politics International* and called "Transactional analysis and our philosophical premises: 70 years on" (Minikin, 2020).

2

THE PREMISE OF ALIENATION

In the 1960s, my father was writing about the formation of Pakistan after colonialism and what had become in the years preceding; a violent partition of India. I expect my father had been traumatised by what he had witnessed. The ongoing hatred that had fuelled the beginnings of this new country meant he understood the critical significance of rupture to engagement, connection, and belonging for a people. All that could have been mobilising when there is a common cause and a sense of moving towards a more positive future seemed to have been lost. He felt it keenly, I think. A future seemed to be slipping away—one whereby people can feel more in charge of their destiny, where they can experience being heard, having an impact and a sense of unity in that experience of togetherness. Prior optimism had been behind independence from the Raj, yet my father's writing was far from celebratory. Rather, it was born from seeming despair of his witnessing of national and international fragmentation, splitting amongst communities, terrible unresolved conflicts and tensions. He speculated on the influence of ideology, the mindset of the dominant collective, and the destructiveness that can cause to a nation's state of mind. He understood that the departure of the British Raj did not leave a blank canvas. There was far too much to recover from. In the few years post-independence, he reflected on this with significant despondency: "The tendency towards alienation is marked and I was brought to wonder if independence has meant any more to the Pakistan people than the substitution of brown raj for British raj." (Hussain, 1966, p. 167).

I had perceived my journey in thinking about alienation as entirely independent of his mind and his academic career. As mentioned previously, I had become captivated by the ideas from radical psychiatry as I had learnt about them from Keith Tudor. To discover my father had been using the term "alienation" with a different emphasis concerning ideology and international relations was a personal revelation for me. For years I had searched for his book and I finally was able to source a copy just as I completed the first draft of my article on radical psychiatry (Minikin, 2018). The book arrived on Christmas Eve and usually when I first get a book, I open it at random; these were the first couple of sentences I read: "Pakistan has

DOI: 10.4324/9780429289231-3

become a society where the weaning of the individual never takes place. Since the meaning of national experience is lost to him, the alienation of the nation and the individual may become incurable." (Hussain, 1966, p. 40).

It was a shock to see that quite independently of any overt dialogue between us on the subject, I had felt compelled to write about the alienation of individuals in their nations. I had done so from the perspective of being a Westerner in terms of a citizen and psychotherapist. So, there was both a difference and a connection to the work of my father at the time of my birth and infancy. He was writing from the position of his formative life experience in both colonial and post-colonial India and Pakistan. He had never talked about such experiences and thoughts with me until the summer of 2017—the 70th year of India's partition.

Something profound happened as I encountered his mind through his book. I experienced the deep and soulful significance of how and why collective trauma and oppression lives through the subjectivity of its people and why it is so fundamentally important that we find opportunity to reflect, think, and make sense of the challenges facing social and individual relations. Life experience needs to be thought about and the connection to my evolving interest and exploration into a need for greater social consciousness in my work and generally in my life, resonated deeply. Our subsequent exchanges have brought renewed vitality to our bond and having had many challenges in our lifelong relationship, we have now had important experiences of mutual empathy, understanding, and respect in these recent years. He is old and frail now, but fortunately for him and me, at the time of writing this, he still has an active, enquiring, and, at times, passionate mind. So, this chapter begins with a personal anecdote. Through this, I have intended to share the relevance of intergenerational and autobiographical[1] determinates in our choices of how we live, think, and work.

Ideology serves to inform us about the macro state, the frame of reference, and the mass practical and psychological structures that hold the fabric of our mindsets. It helps us understand the limitations of creative and independent thought and it helps me appreciate why disciplines such as social constructivism and the exercise and attempts of deconstruction are so critically important in supporting us with our second philosophical premise in TA—that "people can think". In recent years, I have found myself reflecting on this premise; indeed, hanging on to it perhaps fervently at times. As psychotherapists, counsellors, educationalists, consultants, Transactional Analysts, and all our colleagues in social, political, philosophical, and psychological fields, thinking is our commission—we must think and help others to as well. The premise of alienation is about the opposite. That is, it gives us a theory to understand how and why people's minds are decommissioned and they stop thinking. This is a main premise in this book, to explore how and why this happens and what we might do about it. There are, as I see it, different forms of alienation, from the roots in infant development to the social and political contexts in which we work and live. I also talk about our alienation from the land and our environments in general. Given the task of the psychotherapist is often set in working privately in the consulting room, the draw to consider internal worlds as entirely separate entities is understandable. However, from my position, context is critical and the relational dynamic with it determines how people experience their lives. I start by reviewing the roots of the radical psychiatry movement in Transactional Analysis and then move on to exploring some wider and deeper meanings of alienation.

Macro and Micro Perspectives: What Do We Mean by Alienation?

At the heart of the radical psychiatry movement was the premise that alienation is the cause of social and psychological distress. This is a simple, potent, political, philosophical assertion, that also has some grounding in psychological, sociological, and scientific theories. To remind us of the passionate assertion in radical psychiatry, I come to the key text: "People's troubles have their source not within them but in their alienated relationships, in their exploitation, in polluted environments, in war, and in the profit motive." (Steiner et al., 1975, pp. 3–4).

Alienation as a concept has its roots in Marx's philosophy. The key idea being that capitalist economies promote a sense of estrangement ("*entfremdung*") amongst people. In other words, the ideology behind capitalist economic structures cuts people off from their sense of their humanity; they become disconnected from the meaning of their productivity, from their connection with colleagues, from the land/the environment in general, and all of this affects their capacity to engage in intimate social relationships. Marx suggested that people become objectified by being seen as resources, subjugated to the "higher" goals of the economic establishment (Shaw, 2014). He was interested in the transition from an agriculturally based economy to an industrialised one and how that would influence the mindset of the state and its people. He saw the potential for people to be robbed of meaning in their work and in their lives as they surrendered to what Steiner picks up on as the "profit motive". Marx predicted the objectification of people via the production line where the workers are seen as a "resource", the means to an end which is the basis of how large corporations currently work and define their people.

Despite Marx being exiled from Germany and living in London through the abolition of slavery, his focus remained on the working class, their exploitation and subsequent alienation from production, their environment, and each other. In short: alienation from their humanity. Much as I value his premise, I understand my academic learning as being relationally bound with personal and professional life experience. So, here I lean into a social constructivist perspective. I draw on my identity as the daughter of a man from the Punjab region of India and Pakistan and a mother with roots from a White working-class mining background from the midlands in England. I see myself as rooted in the postcolonial experience. Contributing to my identity is my time living in West Africa during my formative childhood years, and then later on in London and Birmingham in the UK. In addition to my inheritance from my father, I have lived closely to the lives and experiences of Black people in Nigeria and in Birmingham. This has evoked a deep empathy for the Black experience, which, in my view, underpins all of our histories.

My take is that alienation as Marx spoke about it—that is, the political, economic, social, and human estrangement from connection with learning and life started way back—with feudalism and with slavery. Slavery is not only to be understood as a socially and psychologically traumatic event, but it also needs to be understood as the historical base to our current economy. Slavery set up a global economic dependency via the triangular trade. It set up the mindset for imperialism, colonialism, indenture, and the more recent modern-day capitalism. So, the objectification of people as a resource, the structures and processes of exploiting the poor for the gain of the wealthy goes way back. Marx predicted the proletariat would rise up and object and that socialism was the inevitable outcome ... Perhaps it is, perhaps revolution will take longer than he thought, and perhaps there are evolutionary outcomes that are not yet conscious. Or perhaps the "revolution" will be born out of something we cannot yet conceive, something we have not thought about. Marx, for example, did not predict the demise of the planet through global warming or the human capacity to destroy the planet via nuclear disaster. However, we can still come to understand this through drawing on alienation and thinking about resolutions. Having touched on my history, philosophy, and my autobiographical motivations, I turn to how I connect this with my professional learning as a psychotherapist, trained in a Western tradition. This has focused largely on the personal by drawing on theories of infant development and attachment, such as in the seminal book, *Why Love Matters*, by Gerhardt (2004).

Alienation and Infant Development: "Why Love Matters"

Gerhardt (2004) outlines the influence of affection, contact, and responsiveness in the development of the infant. Traditionally, psychotherapy has drawn much from infant observation and even taking at times infant development as the primary source of anxieties, personality development, attachment patterns, disturbance and so on. The traditional mother/baby dyad has epitomised the capacity for responsiveness, empathy, attunement, understanding, intimate and intuitive knowing, and affect regulation. We have learnt that if

17

all this is given in adequate supply, a young child will be raised capable of expecting love, respect, joy in living, joy in contact, having a capacity to love, to trust, to be optimistic of welcome, and to be optimistic that the world will respond to their distress. In other words, a healthy human being, secure and connected with self and others. We understand such a person would have confidence and the resilience to face adversity, temporary misattunements, and even some minimal neglect. Such experiences could be endured rather than being defended against via repression or dissociation, because by and large, the world is a good place.

If we extend this picture of confidence and resilience to see what is happening in the mother's world, we have to assume that like the infant, she was feeling supported in her environment. We could assume that she has known and experienced love, that she is optimistic about her role in mothering, and in her immediate and social environment to support her with this. Perhaps such a mother has an evolved sense of self (Johnson, 2017) because she too was responded to with attunement and connection in her family of origin. Her capacity for joy, love, and contact might go way back through the generations. This narrative of infant development is a valid one, one that informs us as to why contact and love is so important. However, the missing stories here are the ones of context, of deprivation, privation, traumas, discrimination, pressures—relational, social, economic, political—all of which put pressure on whoever is raising this child. It puts pressure on the nursing family (taken from Winnicott's nursing triad) and if we know love matters to the health of our babies and children, what is the responsibility of our social structures, our division of resources, our provision of care? In other words, I am asking, what is our social responsibility in raising our future generations?

From my perspective of social responsibility, I am interested in who gets such support with raising our nation's children. Who are the mothers feeling respected and loved and who are feeling estranged in their personal and social environment? What are the personal and collective histories contributing to the alienation of caretakers? How does this play into internal historical relational patterns, inter- and/or transgenerational trauma? What persistent patterns and expectations in families and society require mothers to be endlessly loving and responsive? Does a departure from this deserve condemnation on the caretaker?

The point I am making is that the capitalist perspective on life can be alienating for a range of families and caretakers. So, whoever is doing the "mothering", according to Western psychotherapists, it is meant to be perfect, private, and resourced almost entirely by one individual. Concessions in UK society have been made to include maternal and paternal leave. Yet this too addresses traditional heterosexual norms and our social support for child rearing requires further reviews.

Alienation From Our Bodies: A Personal Anecdote

When living in Nigeria during the 1960s, I remember being entranced by Nigerian working women carrying their babies on their backs. They had an amazing capacity to swing the baby up, tie them up, pick up containers, absolutely full and heavy calabashes containing food or water, or huge bowls of oranges all balanced on their heads as they went about their business. As a young child, I admired this strength, balance, and dexterity enormously and would often try and emulate and imitate such women with my own props. Another feature worthy of general admiration was the capacity of these mothers to know when their child needed to pee. Often, I would see a woman, container on head still, unwrap her wrapper, release the leg of her baby, who would then produce an impressive arc in mid-air. Once done, the baby was swung back on the back, tied in, and off the pair went. This scene had also caught the eye of my English mother and one day she approached such a working woman and asked: *how did she know when the baby needed to pee?* Apparently, the woman turned, looked at my mother, smiled, and said: *Madam, how can you **not** know?*

Knowing my mother, I can sense that an answer to that question is rather complex. To offer the reader, some clues, my maternal grandmother was raised in a Victorian orphanage, so my grandmother herself had, I imagine, been deprived of the sort of love, holding, and attunement that Gerhard writes about. She died when my mother was pregnant with me, and she was my mother's only family when she met my father. So, I was born to a grieving mother. I doubt my mother had experienced the kind of physical contact and holding that she was witnessing between some of these Nigerian mothers and their babies. I think she watched them as a new phenomenon as, clearly, she was curious about them. Writing this nearly 60 years on, I surprise myself with how I vividly I recall the scenes with those mothers from Nigeria. My fascination of the working women in Nigeria may have penetrated me as a child in a different way from my mother's curiosity. However, I do wonder whether we were both drawn to the scene because of what we had missed in our early relationship with each other. Experiences we have not known may mark our internal landscapes like permanent fault lines that can shake or erupt under duress. I make a link here to my historical interest in the study of geography, which takes me to another area I wish to register—feeling alienated from the land.

Alienation From Our Environments

As a teenager, geography and biology were the subjects at school I felt most attracted to. I loved drawing the diagrams, the maps, and learning about the world and the life around me. Later on, perhaps based on poor advice and personal decisions, I did not pursue the study of environmental biology. Rather, I was pushed towards languages as a way forward for potential employment. However, it was no good—I had little talent in that department. So, I was lucky enough to do badly in my final school exams, which took me down the unexpected path of going through "clearing[2]" and reading for a geography degree when I was 18. That gave me the opportunity to learn about ecology and the interdependence of life in the environment. My engagement with geography focused my mind on the relationship between people and their environment and our interdependence on each other. As a young woman, I went back to "Africa" when I studied geography at Portsmouth. I read about the demographic impact of slavery, of colonialism, and of industrialisation in terms of hindering free movement across Africa. The artificial creation of national boundaries by Europeans ruined many rural communities, some of whom survived by being on the move and following the rains. I learnt about the subsequent desertification across sub-Saharan Africa and the deforestation across all tropical areas way back in 1981. The pace of economic development across the continent of Africa via industrialisation, based on a Western model, led to tremendous disparities between the rich and the poor in many countries. Many, if not most, of the rural areas were left neglected as people migrated to the cities in search of work. This was the key characteristic in the early days of post-colonial Africa. It contributed to a profound dismantling of history and culture—an alienation of identity and an estrangement from the connection and meaning of relationship with the environment. Global industrialisation is now the norm for many of us and, in the UK, urban environments are where most of our working class and poorer immigrant communities live. Many writers, poets, musicians, and other artists have portrayed the alienation of industrialised landscapes that cut people off from their experience of humanity and sense of community. I imagine the reader knows of their own connections here, in terms of the artists or musicians they have found some comfort in, at times of loneliness and despair.

At the time of writing this, our planet is in crisis. The compelling competition of international industrialisation and, I would argue, the capitalist "pandemic" has caught the world in a trap it may never be able to free itself from. Whatever political and humanitarian goodwill may exist across the globe, it cannot rival the thrust of economic competition that depends on industrialisation, capitalism, and international and national travel for trade and people. Our planet is doomed to collapse under the pressure. Much as we may all wish for something different, I personally cannot see this happening in my lifetime. The complex web we have created as an international community is too fraught politically with polarised positions that right now are not being held with enough containment. The COVID-19 pandemic saw air quality improve in Delhi, river pollution improve, and natural life return with vigour in a few places—but only for the short term. Some might argue this was an opportunity to review and plan for the saving of the planet. However, without widespread political and social commitment to such a cause, this was never going to be the priority on the planning agenda—certainly not in my country, the UK. Rather, the anxiety about the economy has seen and will continue to see strategy and tactics designed to get us back to "normal". Normal has in my view meant an alienation from the natural environment, particularly for the poorer factions of society who, by and large, live in cities in the UK and in neglected rural areas in other countries. Having experiences of connection with the natural world is tending to become a privilege of the privileged in richer countries.

At the micro scale, we know that we are hardwired to be in relationship with nature. Yet essential needs under capitalism are more likely to be perceived as getting broadband to everyone than getting everyone to green spaces. Being interested in gardening, I have seen gardens pitched on roofs and walls in recent years, though I notice this only adds to my despair. I find myself wondering—does this merely facilitate the excuse to carry on building? Do such novelties in garden design offer more than a perfunctory nod to the destruction we are facing? Is there a risk of treating a deep-rooted problem with sticking plasters? Continuing the use of online working, as discovered during the pandemic, could be helpful. However, the scope that remote working can help is yet to be seen. Meanwhile, the aviation and automobile industries are crying out to be saved. All of this whilst deemed necessary, cuts us off from the natural world, divorces us from the elements, and instead of seeing for ourselves what is happening in the world around us, we as individuals have little agency to affect the global system. The saving of our planet has to be an international endeavour, one where collaboration is top priority, where powerful people would be commissioned to be radical—not for their own interest but for the subsequent generations. This is unlikely to happen in my view. I fear our sense of alienation is too far gone. If this sounds cynical—the reader would be right. When it comes to the future of our planet, I feel particularly bleak and despairing.

Social and Political Relevance

This economic and political interdependence of nations adds complexity to my generalised sense of feeling overwhelmed. The media and communication channels report on events as and when they arise, and most of us, myself included, are not trained or educated in large-scale international politics or economics. We all try to live within our immediate environments as best we can. So, we get piecemeal information, some of which evokes emotional responses, and these are felt collectively, not simply individually. These constellations of experience constitute various collective "states of mind" and I understand this as providing the environmental backdrop for social and psychological work with people. James Sedgwick (2021), in his recent book, refers to the relevance of contextual difficulties in peoples' lives as "horizontal problems". This is a useful way to consider the depth and breadth of psychological dynamics. As a relational practitioner, I consider context as the environment that might facilitate social and political contact and engagement, as well as the environment that alienates people from their own humanity and life. Our physical and human environments co-exist, and both facilitate and alienate. So, in my view, the environment that people live in is relevant for our social and mental health, and in my work as a psychotherapist, I think it is always relationally bound with their presenting issues.

Case example: Harold

Harold is a local man in his 40 s. He is a carpenter, born and raised in rural mid Devon. He has never left the county he tells me. He smiles as he explains that he doesn't understand women.

"Never have!"

"Interesting!" I say. *"How can you have any hope that I will understand you?"*

He laughs at that. *"Dunno! Maybe you can't!"*

So, he chooses me because I was nearby (geographically speaking) and he comes because he has a broken heart. It appears his girlfriend of six months left him after he beat her in a rage. He cries as he discloses his shame.

The next day, a fairly new supervisee arrives. A woman, who is supportive and empathic; she is working with a young man—John. John's girlfriend is threatening police action after a particularly violent beating.

I am new to this area of the UK, but quickly I learn that the sort of sexual politics I studied in the 1980s and 1990s is still relevant. These two heterosexual men are coming to therapy, perplexed and confused that they are beating their partners and not understanding why. I wonder what new territories I will venture into and how my socio-political interest in misogyny can serve me here? I consider the historical as well as current political and social embodiments of misogyny witnessed from our male Western leaders in recent years. So, in this new situation, it is hard for me to separate what Sedgwick (2021) refers to as vertical and horizontal problems. The relational experiences that have newborn opportunity here is that my client, a man rooted in this red soil of West Somerset and mid Devon, is meeting me, a woman who longs for roots and a place she can really call home. Yet, I cannot avoid bringing in what I have seen of the world as I begin to talk and listen in this community.

Alienation from Society and Recent Social History in the UK

The years leading to my writing this have been volatile in the UK and the wider world. In the UK we have had a government focusing on austerity since 2010. This involved a drastic reduction in public spending which adversely affected social services, the health service, education, and public transport. Simultaneously, there was the Syrian refugee crisis, the attacks in Myanmar, the ongoing crisis of refugees from Africa, and, more recently, from Ukraine. All this alongside some dissatisfaction with the European Union (EU) and Britain's ongoing resistance to European identity was galvanised by populist politicians and their ideology. Regarding the EU, the promise that greater sovereignty might somehow resolve these complex political and social challenges was seductive to many. The argument was convincing in part because of the feelings that are evoked during decades of increasing divisions between rich and poor, north and south (especially London), the educated and the manual labourers. It was helpful for those with a "sovereign" ideology of these challenges to further provoke the anxiety of the already threatened and provide opportunity for mass blame (and therefore projections) on "those foreigners" who, apparently, we were not controlling well enough by having firm enough borders. And so, as fear amongst individuals rises, encounters with authority figures who point to "otherness" provide opportunity for the projection of their anger and hate. It may offer a false comfort as people feel their competence and capacity to influence their lives diminish. Alienation from feelings, potential losses, and alienation from "otherness" mounts to a generalised alienation from humanity and potentially a split from a general sense of integrity. This takes me back into our minds and how the social and the psychological are bound.

In the UK, the capacity to exploit "them and us" in recent years has been facilitated by anxiety over hardship, which, it seems to me, is exploited by the powerful. The experience of feeling threatened by outsiders has been fuelled by policies of austerity. This seems to magnify social aggression and envy of those that do "have". In the West, such envy facilitates a narcissistic consumerist culture, which in my lifetime seems to have become an economic and social norm. Our celebrity culture, get-rich-and-famous-quick schemes, and aspirations for beauty and lifestyle serve to alienate by splitting the individual from society, which amalgamates as a split of mind from body. It is an area that has been written about by many:

> When the balance between individual and society breaks down, we can expect cataclysmic disturbances where regression to more regressive or 'debased' (Bion) states of mind takes place ... I suggest that fascism within the mind and within society is the alienated child of this broken marriage.
>
> (Wieland, 2015, p. 12)

Here, Wieland links fascism with alienation. She is writing about a loss of connection that is painful and needs to be defended against. As she explores the breakdown of relationship between the individual and society, I understand that she describes how qualities such as self-sufficiency are idealised. This leads to the primacy of the state and its entitlement to dominance being justified, fought for, and defended. In contrast, democracy is seen as "weak" and ultimately harmful to the state. This validates the rhetoric of strength in nationalism whilst diminishing and dismissing economic, social, and political fallibility or vulnerability. My interpretation is that this promotes "one mind thinking" and is a denigration of philosophical, social, political, and psychological differences. Many democracies support governance and decision-making through majority votes. To my mind, these are always a compromise and seem to bring relief, as if debate and the dialogue this brings can finally be put to an end because "the people have spoken". The risk being a promotion of narrow-minded thinking that assumes "the people" are of "one voice". One voice can only mean one social and cultural context and identity, one gender that is somehow fixated at that moment in time with no room for manoeuvre. Keval (2016) puts this eloquently: "narrow mindedness is also experienced as totalitarian thinking, which permits only one opinion, as in one party politics with no room for rival thoughts and feelings that might express differences of any kind" (Keval, 2016, p. 22).

I read this as describing how "otherness" in society and within the mind is either killed off or banished to the recesses to promote an illusion of strength and certainty. It is as if the masculine and all that might represent has to be aggrandised to protect against the risk that anything representing the feminine can make itself known. And this is grounded in a White racist form of masculinity. For instance, Frantz Fanon writes, "black is not a man" (1952/2021, p. 138), and Wieland (2015) describes the Jews being portrayed as a feminised man in 19th century Germany and across Europe. I think the mode of this sort of dialogue has been revisiting us in some recent political rhetoric in the West, which has given us current day observable examples of what Wieland and Keval discuss in their books. For me, both writers compel the reader to reflect on encounters with these rigid inflexible parts in ourselves and others, and it seems important to recognise how such destructive psychological processes get triggered in our professional, social, and intimate relations. Hence, I suggest social and political expressions mirror reflections of the internal states of people and vice versa. When the relational connection of these break down, I suggest we risk psychic and cultural death.

The Role of the Psychotherapist

Essentially, the role of a psychotherapist is to help people become more conscious so they may feel better about themselves and their relationships. Most of us are trained to work at the micro rather than the macro level—what Sedgwick (2021) refers to as vertical processes. This means that what may come first to the mind of therapists are not the ways in which their clients are alienated but rather a frame of reference about individual ways that "dysfunction" has developed within their family. Sometimes their culture may be used to add or explain historical influences on their state of mind.

Initially, the task of the therapist is often to help clients raise their awareness about their experience. Consciousness is relevant because many people do not understand why they are in a state of distress and that in itself causes pain. People usually are aware they have had stressful life events and that these events have brought them to therapy. However, there is a lot to understand about how these events have affected their mind, body, and soul, let alone what might need to happen to alleviate that distress. Different disciplines will disagree about the best way to approach these problems and help people with them. However, all practitioners are engaged in the same endeavour—how to help people with their state of mind. I believe that the difficulty within people lies in their experiences of relational, social, political, and/or cultural alienation. Furthermore, when processes of their "horizontal" trauma (Sedgwick, 2021) are positioned as an individual ("vertical") process, I believe that the therapist risks retraumatising their patient. I make this point because in these circumstances, the therapist unwittingly misses the existence or significance of how the social, economic, and/or political experience is alienating their patients.

In outlining my interpretation of social and political events, I aim to reveal how I think relationally about our connections and disconnections with our environments. These include our imagination based on life experiences that create constellations of experience and meaning in our minds. I propose that Transactional Analysts and all professionals working with the social and psychological are bound to be profoundly affected by their history, their subjective constellations, and the learning they have received within their training and how it is relationally bound with previous and current life experiences. Hence, it is inevitable that my subjectivity including my political perspectives will make relational contact in my work with clients, supervisees, and trainees. We worry of course that we become oppressive if we push our perspectives on to others and we wish to avoid misusing our power. However, this is not about telling clients how they should cast their vote. It is about staying alive to the process of thinking. As psychotherapists, we position ourselves as willing to use our minds in the service of others as well as to be willing to reflect and think on their perspectives so that we stretch as best we can from dogmatism to democracy. This is the way I think about working at depth and working with the edges of consciousness to deepen and expand minds. In the next chapter, I continue with exploring both the macro and micro perspectives when it comes to the experiences of oppression. As named in Chapter One, oppression is a part of the dynamics that contributes to alienation.

Notes

1 Keith Tudor (personal communication, November 12, 2002) also once said that all theory was autobiographical, and his words have returned to me many times since I developed my thinking on alienation.
2 In the UK, "clearing" is the process by which students who did not get the grades to enter the university of their choice can apply for any other course or place where there are spaces.

3

OPPRESSION

Given the centrality of alienation to my philosophy, I anticipated that writing this chapter on oppression would be the most straightforward one. However, the experience of sitting down at the keyboard proved me wrong. This has been the most challenging part of my writing to date. I struggled to know where to start—with my mind, "the mind" in general, with particular mind-sets, with societies as I witness and experience them, or with entire political countries? The overwhelm within my mind was escalating into chaos. In an effort to contain my process, I turned to a number of dictionary definitions, looking for a way forward that would help me manage to think about, grasp and explore the experience of oppression in a meaningful way. In essence, there were references to areas, regions being shattered, destroyed, killings taking place, unfair and cruel treatment of people, misplaced and overuse of authority and so on. I was struck by the violent language and images of decimation and with this in mind, I started to write.

Shattered Regions

The image that impacted me as I read some of the definitions was one of regions under siege, followed by images of war leaving devastation and trauma. In the first draft of this chapter, I had been flooded with such pictures, particularly of countries I knew about and had a connection with. In the first draft of this chapter, I thought of India, Pakistan, Bangladesh, and Myanmar. Then Nigeria and moving to other countries in Africa—Rwanda, Zimbabwe, Eritrea, South Africa, and then others, including the recent devastating war in Ukraine. All this came flooding in. I moved to the Middle East, to Israel, Palestine, Syria. I kept returning to Syria and a memory I have of asking my father about Syria when we, in the UK, had first heard of their difficulties. My father shook his head saying, "*Syria is very complicated*". As I attempted to collect my thoughts for this chapter, I spent several days researching Syria, poring over photo-graphs of bomb-shattered Damascus. The reader will not know that, during the 1990s, I had many opportunities to visit Syria. I was captivated by the ancient city of Damascus. It got into me somehow and remains one of the

DOI: 10.4324/9780429289231-4

most memorable cities I had ever been to. The city is more than 8000 years old, and everywhere I looked I seemed to see and feel the centuries of meaningful experiences of the people who had lived and walked there before me. Later, to see photographs of the devastation was terrible, haunting. Perhaps by way of trying to process something, I sent the editor of this book a series of photographs of Damascus—before and after the devastation. As I come now to review this chapter, I am preoccupied by what is happening right now in Ukraine. I have never visited this country but have known colleagues and friends from the region. This is a country with which many of us have professional and personal connections and so the traumas are close, and the pictures and stories horrifying. Just as with the other war-torn countries I have mentioned, people will be haunted by what has happened for generations to come. When it came to my first draft of the book, I realised that in trying to write about Syria, I was reaching out beyond my means and scope. So, I put the first draft of this chapter in the bin.

It was nine months before I returned to face it again. I have no idea if this was gestation, material formulating during that time, or whether I was simply avoiding feeling overwhelmed again. I had considered abandoning this entire project, convincing myself that it was getting too late for a book like this and perhaps what I was trying to do was all too much like hard work at this stage of my life. So, I struggled to gather my mind and thoughts. "Regions under siege, images of war, devastation and trauma". I had been searching the external, the real "regions under siege", whilst also realising that these external experiences mirror the internal landscapes of our minds, the inner experience of being and feeling "under siege".

Returning to the chapter I realised with humility and some humour that my job was not simply to over-identify with all those places shattered by oppression in a way that rendered me incapacitated, but that I was to keep exercising some capacity to think and reflect on what it all might mean. What does it mean for me, my clients, and the specific contexts that have helped shape them? How can the dictionary definition of oppression be useful or relevant? I live a pretty safe and secure life after all. Working mainly in the UK, I question the extent to which I encounter the kind of cruelty, injustice, or authoritarianism that some nations are subject to. It is important to emphasise the obvious in that many people do endure actual situations of serious and ongoing oppression. As we saw with the death of George Floyd, some people suffer within a so-called "liberal and free" state and we also know that in many other nations and areas persecution of whole groups of people is much more manifest. This is different from the psychological oppression we can all experience where conscious or unconscious processes collaborate to diminish or kill off parts of our subjective experiences or part selves. In therapeutic work, I think we have been slow to recognise the psychological impact of social neglect, discrimination, and day-to-day trauma. We have been short-sighted in how these dynamics have been taught, facilitated, and worked with clinically. In part, this has reflected our institutions that struggle to see a wide range of social representation in qualified practitioners and struggle to know how to integrate the political with the psychological. So, recently, we have been playing catch-up and Black authors (for example, Mckenzie-Mavinga, 2016; Ellis, 2021; Turner, 2021) have been commissioned to help us do this.

There is a need to account for the real social threat to visibility and existence in the consulting room. It needs accounting for in a way that raises consciousness and can position responsibility where it belongs. The fact that some people will continue to live in an unequal and oppressive situation after having counseling or psychotherapy also needs to be thought about. Sometimes our enthusiasm and faith in our theories can evoke an unrealistic sense of what is possible, and this in itself can be reflective of privilege and reinforce oppression. The global pandemic experience was another way whereby enormous inequality within and between societies was exposed.

At the time of rewriting this chapter, Ukraine is under siege, and England has moved out of lockdown. The UK is failing to report the ongoing burden that the National Health Service (NHS) is still carrying. Brexit and its consequences rumble on. The G7 has long completed its conference in Cornwall, where it seems little was achieved. The United States and its new president attempt to repair some national and international damage, and the echoes of the George Floyd killing reverberate alongside the many other unarmed Black people killed at the hands of police (Quah & Davis, 2015). Situated here in England, I am subjected to more news from Europe and the United States than the rest of the world, so this in itself will be shaping my frame of reference and the resources I have at hand to help me think. I, like others, need to occasionally see and hear others having similar thoughts. This can feel sustaining and supportive, re-sourcing us to face the ongoing stretch of challenging our thinking and emotional states in the work that we do. I describe the efforts it may take to hold on to a mind sufficiently enough to be able to think, feel, and reflect on our lives and our leaders, to hold ethical integrity, to feel part of a community, and to have a sense of some agency. To do all these things, we need the support of others too, especially when we live in a context that is oppressive.

As I thought about the situation in the UK, with the pandemic and with mental health in general, I was drawn to investigate a little further. Instead of photographs of Damascus, I started poring over statistics related to mental health in the UK. The figures, in this next section, are taken before the pandemic of 2020–2021.

The impact of mental ill health

- 1 in 4 people experience mental health issues each year.
- At any given time, 1 in 6 working-age adults have symptoms associated with mental ill health.

- Mental illness is the second-largest source of burden of disease in England. Mental illnesses are more common, long-lasting and impactful than other health conditions.
- Mental ill health is responsible for 72 million working days lost and costs £34.9 billion each year. Note: Different studies will estimate the cost of mental ill health in different ways. Other reputable research estimates this cost to be as high as £74–£99 billion.
- People with a long-term mental health condition lose their jobs every year at around double the rate of those without a mental health condition. This equates to 300,000 people—the equivalent of the population of Newcastle or Belfast.
- Men aged 40–49 have the highest suicide rates in the UK.
- 70–75% of people with diagnosable mental illness receive no treatment at all.
- In an average classroom, ten children will have witnessed their parents separate, eight will have experienced severe physical violence, sexual abuse or neglect, one will have experienced the death of a parent and seven will have been bullied (MHFA England, 2020, para. 2).

The third bullet point states: "Mental illness is the second-largest source of burden of disease in England. Mental illnesses are more common, long-lasting and impactful than other health conditions" (MHFA England, 2020, para. 2).

These figures startled me and contributed to the stalling in my process that I described earlier. I had no idea what I could write about that as the statement speaks for itself. So, continuing the theme of needing to make something huge manageable, I took on "the second largest burden of disease", "more common, long-lasting and impactful than any other health condition". Considering this further, I decided to say something about the state of our mental health provision in the UK. I am grateful for the insights offered by Dalal (2018) in his extraordinary book, *CBT: The Cognitive Behavioural Tsunami*, which is thoroughly researched and taught me a great deal.

Twenty years ago, the UK was governed by "Labour". Traditionally this had been the political party that represented the working population of the UK—the ordinary people, so to speak. Richard Layard was a Labour minister who had recognised the scale of the problem regarding mental health. Quoted as the "godfather of CBT" (Bion, 1959), he is described as a neoliberal rationalist who has reduced mental distress to a problem that simply has to be solved: "The inner life … determine[s] how we react to life … So how can we gain control over our inner life?" (Layard, 2005, p. 184).

Logic, the rational mind, and the capacity for cognitive control points to a "mastering" of feelings, as distress seems to be problematic. So, if distress leading to depression is the problem with rationality and control being the solution, we can see how Cognitive Behavioural Therapy (CBT) has come to be attractive to ministers, mostly men who have some responsibility and authority over an escalating social problem. CBT is the dominating force for "treatment" supported by the medical system in the UK. In addition to Dalal's passionate critique of the influx of CBT, the "siege" of it so to speak, I wish to emphasise that this frame of reference is embedded in the masculine. Hence, my use of the word "mastering" was deliberate. Dealing with depression and anxiety through eradicating vulnerability is in line with the "manufacturing of masculinity" (Wieland, 2015) described in the previous chapter. I think this has compounded the problems of mental health provision in the UK. My argument is supported by evidence of the overtly sexist argument in the crude use of a rational, "logical" explanation offered by Layard for the cited increase in depression amongst women:

> Women whose pay and opportunities have improved considerably relative to men, but whose level of happiness has not ... perhaps women now compare themselves more directly with the men than they used to and therefore focus more than before on the gaps that still exist.
>
> (Layard, 2005, as cited in Dalal, 2018, p. 45)

This seems to point to the need to keep facts about inequality away from the minds of those who are oppressed by injustice lest they become depressed about it! Following the "ignorance is bliss" argument, there is a profound sense of threat in a neoliberal mindset of the raising of consciousness. Consciousness it seems can cause depression, distress, disturbance, and despair. Awareness of inequalities, of power and privilege, are not good, or so it would seem for the illusion of emotional wellbeing and our "mental health". In Layard's argument, there is also a suggestion that when opportunities are offered, the other should be grateful and happy that their lot in life has improved. Furthermore, the pointing of responsibility upon the women for using their minds to compare absolves the men from having had more than their fair share of resources for years and acting in ways that have maintained this unfair situation. The sickness therefore resides in the women and what it seems they need is some sort of masculine cure.

I now turn to how our formal and informal communications include the social/cultural and political contexts we have known and lived with. How do our interactions contribute to defences, enactments, as well as healing in our work? What are the extra dimensions that relational connection offers for the dynamics of oppression within alienation? To facilitate this, I turn to one of the core ideas in Transactional Analysis. That is Transactional Analysis "proper", and "rules" of communication.

"Rules" or Bridges in Communication?

Berne (1961) presented many ideas that had clarity, and he based these on a deep study of how people operate, communicate, and relate to each other.

One of these ideas appearing in his first book was "rules of communication". In short, he identified three rules:

1 Complementary Transactions. Here, there is a sense of conversational flow … that the message offered from one person is received in the intended way by the other.
2 Crossed Transactions. This serves as the opposite effect of complementary. Here, the state of mind addressed is not the one that responds.
3 Ulterior Transactions: Berne acknowledged that there is often more than one message when we communicate and that the psychological level of the message will determine the outcome of the transaction.
4 In 2005, Novellino added a fourth rule: "The result of unconscious communication depends on the therapist's intuitive ability to decode the psychological level of the transferential transaction" (Novellino, 2005, pp. 168–169).

Berne mapped his "rules" of communication onto his diagrams of ego states, showing clearly how moment-by-moment transactions work. At this point, it is worth commenting on the term, "rules" (C. Shadbolt, personal communication, May 13, 2022). It denotes authority, hard reality, a fact—not to be questioned, examined, or discussed. It is reflective of a "one person" psychology (Stark, 1999), indicative of practice in the middle of the 20th century. The theory shows the keen attention Berne paid to detail, and his observations of what happens in communication are thought provoking and useful. However, the application of how to help relatedness and the context of the process were not part of his analysis. Paying attention to these may add some value to what he noted. For instance, in a crossed transaction, the theory states that one or both parties need to change ego state for communication to continue, but Berne did not illustrate how this was influenced by factors in the environment or show the reader how this was achieved. Neither did Novellino illustrate how the therapist comes to *intuit*, comes to know. Neither Berne nor Novellino really accounted for how to navigate these different minds and different contexts. Novellino implied the therapist needs to be available in the moment with a capacity to read the transferential transaction. Rather than having to see the process spontaneously, in the moment as it were, in a different way, Shadbolt (2012) described how meaning can be arrived at via willingness, relatedness, and tenacity to make contact even though there is an experience of not knowing. By being courageous to enter the uncertain space, to hold openness and dialogue, Shadbolt shows how a crossed transaction could be worked with and how to establish engagement after a rupture—how to move towards a decoding of the psychological transaction. Following the relational endeavour while accounting for context and alienation also helps us to widen our lens and consider how to build bridges when two different minds and different contexts collide. One way of thinking about this in terms of transference and transactions is, "the *content* of transference is usually related to infantile patterns while the *intensity* is the result of the patient's alienation" (Fromm, 1962/2009, p. 41).

Systemic Perspectives on Communication

Thinking about the role of alienation in communication including transferential dynamics allows us to consider the power relations within and between us. In thinking more about the systemic perspective and the theory of alienation, I suggest that complementary transactions require a connection, a mutual understanding sometimes from similar frames of reference. It may be that this could represent a power-sharing dialogue where both parties enjoy connections, mutuality, and engagement. In contrast, complementary transactions could also indicate a collusion with systemic oppression. For example, *we both know what we are talking about and neither do we need to rock our systemic boat.* In other words, the oppression from the oppressor is received and responded to by the oppressed. The oppression is accepted out of a sense of needing to survive and/or belong. The status quo continues—there is an absence of conflict or tension, and there may even be a sense of actual or deluded peace.

When it comes to crossed transactions, perhaps Berne was pointing to an interpersonal misunderstanding, or an outright conflict between two people. Taking this to a systemic perspective is the possibility of a protest to the oppression. This could indicate the emerging of conflict from awakening consciousness. Berne added that the communication in this scenario is jarred or broken, and one or more parties will need to shift for communication to continue. Thinking about the oppression + deception formula, we could assume that something disruptive to the message of oppression has occurred here and acceptance cannot be assumed. So, for dialogue to continue, a process of negotiation or diplomacy would need to be activated; one or both parties have to move position. Something psychically, practically, or socially needs to happen.

The third "rule" or "bridge" in communication has been critical in psychotherapy. We are trained to listen and work with the implicit. In other words, what lies beyond the words. Hence, when Berne states that the outcome of the transaction will be determined at the psychological level, he means that the feelings evoked by the communication are more important than the words. He was keen to expose the unconscious dynamics in games, the psychological transactions, and the deceptions in our communication. Novellino took this a step further by promoting the significance of the unconscious and the need for the therapist to listen to that, hear it, and be capable of putting words to that which has not been spoken. So, Novellino emphasised there was something else to think about: the capacity of the practitioner and the influence this has on the direction the work can take. I argue that in marrying the relational with the radical we can begin to account for internal and external worlds and how they serve to influence connections and disconnections with each other. Contexts will include power dynamics that operate within and between people and therefore contribute to the nature and development of our conversations with each other. So, how might this manifest interpersonally and institutionally in psychotherapy?

Returning to the access to psychotherapy in the UK, if people are distressed enough by life events and if these "out there" experiences evoke the internalised state of depression or anxiety, they might be "lucky" enough to be admitted for a course of CBT offered by our National Health Service. Treatment encourages them to be rational, to examine the illogicality of their state of mind. In other words, to set up a binary competition between the rational and irrational. This is, of course, in aid of reducing symptoms as opposed to the endeavour of becoming known to oneself and to others. It is possible that there may be a case for this being a good option for some patients in some situations. However, the prescription risks a furthering of alienation of people from their internal life, from their emotional world, and from experiences of being related to. Patients are taught to decommission their feelings, eradicate their vulnerability, and defeat their subjectivity by aligning with objective thought. Figuratively speaking, and drawing from the symbolic world, it seems to pursue a triumph of the conscious rational mind over the possibility of making further links (Bion, 1959) and connections through mentalising affect (Fonagy et al., 2002). However, that is a potential triumph for those who actually manage to be successful patients. The research and randomised control trials in the UK have become possible because of the large numbers of people seen through this scheme. The results seem to indicate people benefit and there is a reduction of symptoms. Nonetheless, despite the massive IAPT (Improving Access to Mental Health Provision) Project[1] that Layard and Clark pioneered to privilege short-term CBT treatment for mood disorders, the mental health situation in the UK continues to be terrible, national figures are not at all improved, and I imagine are likely to be much worse after the pandemic. The plans going forward under this current government cite some additional provision for young people and perinatal women, but point to ongoing increasing support and provision of the IAPT service (NHS, 2019).

The analysis by Dalal (2018) is an eye-opener in terms of socio-political power and how it is used with an enormous institution such as the NHS. The support for a medical model, a modern Western scientific mindset about mental health, is embedded in the very fabric of our national mental health provision in the UK. It has supported a split in the profession whereby diversity of philosophies, theories, and approaches are just about tolerated as long as they remain marginalised on the fringes of provision via the private sector, but not validated, recognised, or given any clout by the mainstream.

The psychological education system implemented in the UK continues to maintain the institutional and systemic oppression around how we think about vulnerability, and the system continues to keep opportunities and access to mental health provision profoundly unequal. So, there is a long way to go before vulnerability to anxiety, depression, and/or substance abuse is analysed and thought about in more systemic and humane ways. There is insignificant consideration paid to how we organise our communities, our resources, and our responsiveness. Perhaps it all feels too much. We are all so immersed in our systemic worlds that trying to step out of such a mindset proves utterly overwhelming. Borrowing words from Mark Fisher (2009): "Capitalism is what is left when beliefs have collapsed at the level of ritual or symbolic elaboration, and all that is left is the consumer–spectator, trudging through the ruins and the relics" (p. 4).

The capitalist engulfment has to my mind penetrated the fabric of our systems, institutions, and states of mind and so it is unsurprising that in the West our dominant approach to mental health supports the CBT frame. Defined as a "tsunami" by Dalal, it has created a particular mindset around mental health that will, in my view, take generations to change.

Case example: Alan

Alan was a builder. He had just had his first child and he came to see me because he couldn't stop crying. Both his parents had been dependent on alcohol, and he had suffered personal, social, and educational neglect. During his teenage years he was diagnosed with severe dyslexia which had explained his earlier struggle with reading and writing. However, by then he had given up on school. He had survived the humiliation of several teachers by becoming a classroom joker. This won him a few friends and saved him from fights with the bigger and stronger boys. At school, he told me he made friends with the Black kids and the "weird" kids, so he reported. When he went home, he and his sister made jam sandwiches. He took a friend home from school one day and as he turned into his house, his mother was lying collapsed on the doorstep—door open. He said he simply "stepped over her". I could see and feel the deep contempt on his face as he recalled that memory. He and his sister had been two of those children who fell in between the cracks of the social care system and survive in families that are poor by UK standards and suffering themselves, no doubt, from generations of neglect. In January 2021, 1% of the UK population owned 25% of the wealth (Savage, 2021) and people like Alan are common. Despite this depressing backdrop, there was some attachment in the family and some camaraderie between him and his sister—enough to get by, and he had managed to get work in the hospital and to have a steady partner.

35

Now Alan was a father, he was unravelling and finding it difficult to cope with life. We could understand this as a recycling of his early childhood and the possible overwhelm his under-resourced parents may have felt. This would have ill-equipped him for his own experiences of fatherhood. However, it was not the whole story and the socio-economic situation he was in as an infant, a child, and now as a new parent has also been accounted for. Having previously worked as a porter in a mental hospital, he had known that there were counsellors and psychotherapists and so he came to me—a White working-class man, looking for someone to help him. He was available because he was broken, desperate, and full of feelings of failure as a man. So, what is the therapeutic task when someone like Alan appears at our doorstep? In what ways is oppression at work around and within him?

Alan: "Prolonged cruel or unjust treatment"

With reference to Alan, I have described his experiences of alienation via his social class, his educational trauma, and the frequent abandonments his parents inflicted on him via their addiction to alcohol. The oppression he experienced was of being robbed of dignity, integrity, and being left vulnerable to blame and bullying by some teachers and pupils at his school. In the wider social realm, there was a lack of role models from his background—a lack of people like him being respected who could guide him. These disadvantages in life meant he struggled for resources which limited the choices that were available to him. His parents were also oppressed people who had not been helped with their social or psychological alienation and so were getting through the stresses in life via the bottle. The potential deceptions that rendered the oppression unconscious was held as his script system—that, somehow, he was to blame for everything in his suffering, that he was stupid, that his parents were incompetent, and that he buys into the lack of respect for men like him and believes he is indeed unworthy.

This is not to say that in my way of thinking Alan was simply an innocent victim of the oppressive system. Rather, thinking about "radical reformation" (Minikin, 2018), I aim to acknowledge, account for, and work with the impact of the system getting in and shaping his mind, which gets reinforcing evidence from the normative structures and processes within society that there is something fundamentally wrong with his basic human value. In other words, his dignity and his humanity are flawed.

When people are humiliated, they are robbed of dignity, and I described how Alan reported this to me. He had introjected his experience of falling short of others' expectations, he had talked about the shame he felt for being inadequate in some way, and he went on to talk to me about the humiliation he felt as a man when he could not respond to seductive moves from his wife. Physically, psychically, and sexually he felt impotent.

His treatment at school robbed him of confidence in his capacity to think—his ability to trust his own mind. To trust one's own mind we have to be in a position to take ourselves seriously, which includes taking our feelings seriously. How is such a thing possible if vulnerability (perhaps especially in men) has to be eradicated. These forms of oppression point to the "manufacturing of masculinity" (Wieland, 2015) which, as I have argued, is a normative frame of reference permeating structures, processes, policies, debate, and psychologies certainly still here in the UK, in the West, and no doubt many other areas of the world. All of this—the measure, or what it is to be good, to be respected, to be valued, to have a place, to be somebody—all of this was permeating Alan's mind. Picking up on these themes, I consider how oppression leads to the experience of being marginalised in society, for men like Alan, as well as for people with other forms of marginalised identities.

Oppression and Social Marginalising

Since the murder of George Floyd, there has been a stirring in consciousness about systemic racism. This has inspired a greater awareness of how oppression works at the macro level. However, the psychological and social adaptation to an oppressive state of mind cannot be underestimated. Under stress, the systemic gets a grip. One recent example from the UK comes from a campaign by a footballer. Football is a game for the people and Marcus Rashford is a Black English footballer. In 2021, he was playing for Manchester United and England. During the pandemic, he campaigned along with chef Tom Kerridge (Butler, 2021) that children from the poorest families in the UK would benefit from one wholesome meal a day. For his work, he was awarded recognition from the Queen and given an MBE (Member of the British Empire)[2]. His campaign was worthwhile, and he stuck to it with tenacity, even when our government pushed back. The fact that our government pushed back is perhaps some indication of how we found ourselves in this position in the first place. How come we have families and children in poverty in the UK? This is a question not just for us, but for the world. It is within our capability to ensure that all children in this world are fed well. They are not because of our systemic structures and processes that continue to support disparities in wealth. Although there are altruistic arguments that support the capitalist quest, these forces across nations do not exist or thrive in order to make money to look after the vulnerable. The vulnerable and those that support them usually must fight to get enough. This is because despite what might be said, contempt (in my view) exists for those that have a need. Marcus Rashford was intermittently a hero; an important spokesperson for ordinary people that struggled. Then in May 2021, his team lost an important game. In reaction, some fans turned on him with racial abuse.

People are quick to feel thwarted and robbed—of success or even a state of mind that they feel entitled to have. This helps people avoid or defend against loss. So, the anger with grief can get projected outwards in expressions of hate and the people that are meant to pick this up and hold it are the marginalised in society. Being a Black hero is precarious because one's sense of being somebody, someone who can be respected for taking a stand, having a strong moral purpose, speaking out with independent mind—all of this stands on vulnerable ground and one's visibility for achieving can also lead to a visibility that makes one the target of attack. This is how I understood the racial abuse hurled at Rashford because his team dared to lose. Winning would protect him temporarily from hate—but as a Black man, he has no doubt had to live the reality that hate is never far away. Talking about Ebony Rainford-Brent, the first Black woman cricketer to play for England in 2007, Michael Holding states how she endured appalling racial abuse throughout her career. Speaking out in 2020, she then withdrew, for fear of the backlash:

> She has suffered. It has affected her health and it had a profound impact on her career. It is such a tragedy that Black people can't even go to their jobs, where they excel, where they want to achieve and want to thrive, without having to put up with this … she has withdrawn from the conversation, fearing a backlash because she dared to say something. She is afraid. Women, whatever the context always seem to suffer more. They are considered targets for particularly vile abuse.
>
> (Holding, 2021, pp. 15–16)

Is it any wonder therefore that people who are Black, who identify as gay or trans, who are neurodiverse, or live with disability may encounter more complex challenges with their mental health? They are pushed by society to hold vulnerability—to be projected on to, to be undermined and robbed of resources. Of course, they will as a result be more vulnerable. Here are two statements from the same report about mental health in the UK that I quoted earlier:

- Young people from BAME [Black, Asian and minority ethnic] and migrant backgrounds are more likely to show developmental difficulties associated with psychosis and develop psychotic disorders later in life.
- 11%–32% of young people who identify as LGBT+ have attempted suicide in their lifetime (MHFA England, 2020, para. 2).

The polarisation of masculine versus feminine and strength versus weakness has long been under scrutiny. The binary thinking is being deconstructed and dismantled further by the studies of intersectionality, and with reference to this dimension, contemporary gender and sexual identity politics throws down a powerful gauntlet. For men like Alan, a man raised in the masculine rhetoric of our parents and fore-parents, he was afflicted by the claustro-phobic pressure of what, who, and how he had to be to be a man. His history and class had already put him on the back foot, and the strain of his eco-nomic and social history and the impact this had on his parents were taking their toll on him. The introjection of his parents, and their social and eco-nomic oppression was all identified with and defended against with mas-culine fortitude, but the tension could not hold, and the chains of this entrapment were broken. We had to see what we could salvage in the wreckage. Luckily for us, he was broken but not decimated. He still had a capacity to think and so we had something to work with.

Alan was a man that knew the oppression of feeling like a failure. In all sorts of ways—his neglect, his social class, and his lack of academic support all played into a sense that he was not a "winner" in life (see Berne's, 1972, "winning scripts").

In terms of masculinity as a construct, "otherness" as a man in society and within one's mind gets killed off or banished to the recesses to promote an illusion of strength and certainty. It is as if the masculine and all that it might represent has to be identified with, and aggrandised to protect against the risk that anything representing vulnerability can make itself known. This is grounded in the White racist form of masculinity that I mentioned in Chapter Two.

For Alan, I knew his family container—his intergenerational inheritance included a struggle with poverty within the context of the UK, his social container included the British denigration of working people, and his ex-istential reality was that he had just become a parent. He was struggling enormously with this responsibility given the fallibilities in his mind and sense of self which had been afflicted from the social and psychological oppression socially, as well as parental neglect.

In my work, it was apparent that he struggled daily and deeply with a profound sense of inadequacy, of "Bad Me" (if I draw on Sullivan, 1953). Hence, I suggest social and political expressions influence the internal states of people through provision of the relational container. When relational connec-tion breaks down, I suggest we risk psychic and cultural demise—even death. The latter relates to dissociative, disavowed experiences, the sense of which can only be recognised if it resides outside of the self, or as Sullivan described, "Not Me".

In Transactional Analysis, we can think of "Bad Me" (Sullivan, 1953) representing our experiences of ourselves in script—the parts our counter script wishes to protect us from. As a working man, Alan had been invested in a bravado kind of counter script. We could call that "Be Strong" in TA. Such a counter script helped keep his vulnerability at bay. We know that the counter script cannot always hold because it is not the whole story—it is not the truth of who we are. Given enough pressure and enough provocation, the psyche will drop into the place it has been dreading. "Bad Me" is the identification we have of ourselves that we know but don't like. Alan was very ashamed of his vulnerability, of feeling stupid, inadequate, of feeling impotent as a man. He had begun to drink as a way of coping with his overwhelm and was very frightened of repeating patterns from his parents and his own history—much was his fear, and much was his shame. His struggle with drinking to try and cope added to his feelings of shame and was an attempt to protect himself from disintegrating further into a sense of utter worthlessness. This terror was pointed to a fragmented state of mind that could not hold a plural sense of self. The threat of vulnerability to his identity as a man was utterly devastating. Hence, vulnerability and manhood could not be linked. I argue this was a divided mindset that also reflected social processes: "The disavowal of those deemed the most socially abject is not exclusively a racial, or a colour, matter. It runs through the social relations of class, gender, sexuality and intimacy" (Hall, 2017, p. 102).

Script Protocol and Enactments: "Not Me"

I consider that our ancestral legacy is reflected in our script protocol. In Transactional Analysis, script protocol goes to the roots, or the bedrock of what underpins our defences. This is the legacy of the deeply unprocessed material in our parents that we experience through our bodies in contact with them. Their bodies and our bodies are affected by what contains them and us as we come into being. Their dysregulated feelings are felt and become ours to deal with or not. Fragmented experiences and contexts that have been overwhelming for them gets passed unprocessed down through the generations and we inherit it all. This is why slavery, colonialism, and indenture matters. It is why Alan's legacy of English class politics matters. His parents found refuge through drinking. The seeking comfort through suckling, ingesting, and hoping that something sustaining will be found, but it never was for them. Alan struggled to find sustaining comfort, stability, or love. His sense of pride in who he was, in his creative capacity, his vitality, and his authentic strength needed bringing to life. This was his "Not Me" self that was yet to be born. I continue his story in Chapter Eight. In the following chapter, I follow on the theme of oppression with the destructive impact this can have for nations and individuals in terms of their relational connection with their identity. I am returning to Africa—the mother of all nations as a way of symbolising how a person and a people can be undermined, dismantled, and then controlled.

Notes

1 An enormous research project that recruited novices and practitioners into a CBT training scheme to provide time focused CBT to patients.
2 The irony that our honours include this wording is not lost on the author.

4

THE COLONISING OF LANDS AND MINDS

"Things Fall Apart"

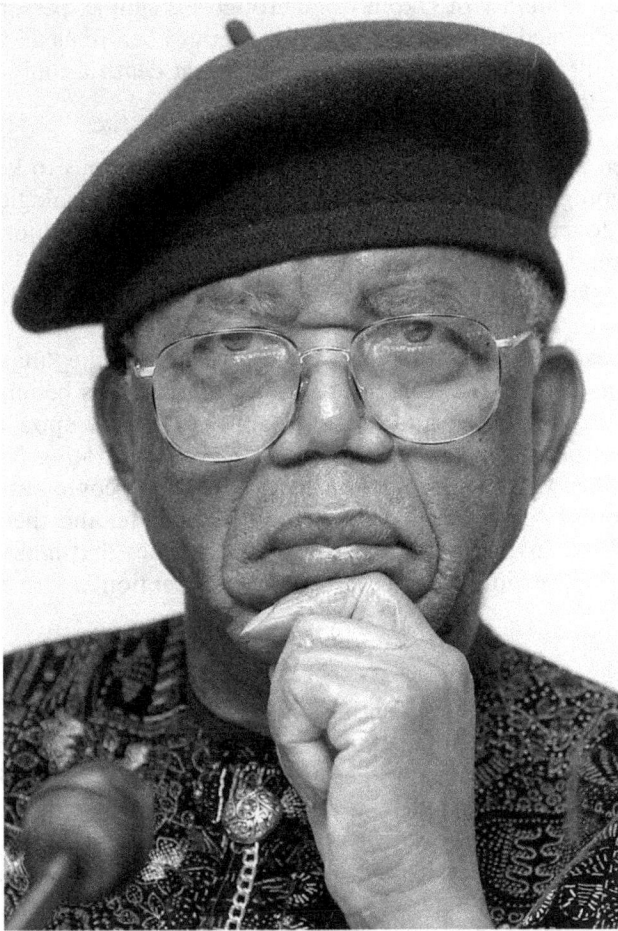

Figure 4.1 Chinua Achebe, Nigerian poet and novelist in 2002, aged 72. (Reproduced with permission from Alamy).

DOI: 10.4324/9780429289231-5

Introduction

I start this chapter by honouring Chinua Achebe, who was born in 1930 in Ogidi, Nigeria. He won an initial scholarship to a government school and then gained another to study medicine, with which he went to a new University College at Ibadan in 1948. Later he switched from medicine to reading English, History, and Religious Studies. Between 1958 and 1964 he wrote four novels. *Things Fall Apart* is the first of these. They are a series that tell personal stories around the time of colonialism and then the subsequent years. This first book describes the demise of traditional Igbo culture because of the arrival of the British as colonisers. The main character is Okonkwo, a respected wrestler and leader in the village. Achebe depicts the values of the people, the structures and processes of the culture, and the pride and anger which were a part of the human fallibility of Okonkwo. Through his simple, personal illustrations, we are invited into a world that disintegrates before us and dies under colonial assault. As Berne (1963) writes, the most death dealing force for a group or organisation is "disruption".

> But even if there are enough people ready and anxious to keep the group going, so that it survives both physically and ideologically, it can be destroyed as an effective force by violating its major group structure. This is called disruption.
>
> (Berne, 1963, p. 68)

This describes the intrusion from outside forces across the "major external boundary" as defined by Berne (1963). If that intruder is better organised, "the centre cannot hold" and "mere anarchy is loosed upon the world" (Yeats, 1919, para. 1). Achebe started his novel by quoting Yeats whose words described what happened not just to the Igbo people but to most of the tribes across Africa. Their values, their way of life, and their social organisation fell apart, and so I explore three dynamics that make the domination from oppression possible. The first is "deception".

Deception

The writing from Steve Biko identifies the psychological intention in gaining power through the mind of the other: "The most potent weapon in the hands of the oppressor is the mind of the oppressed" (Biko, 1978, p.68).

Whether it be promulgated by a political and social system, a cult, or an individual, deception is the deadly component within alienation that allows the oppressor to move in and gain control of the oppressed. The dynamic was well known to Berne and writing back in the 1940s—he thought a great deal about Hitler's rise to power and capacity to drum up mass hysteria and following from society at large. Berne used his psychoanalytical training to try and make sense of something that was so successful, yet so inhumane and mad. He was clearly deeply and profoundly impacted personally, socially, politically, and psychologically by Hitler's rise to power, and he used this as motivation to analyse how such a thing had become possible. Later in life, we know Berne became much quieter politically. However in his book, *The Mind in Action* (Berne, 1947, and also referenced in Berne, 2020), as well as in *The Structure And Dynamics of Organizations and Groups* (Berne, 1963), he described the necessary deception that had to be used to gain such a following:

> An evil leader does all he can to use his power to twist reality, so as to make it appear like the images, he gives his people to go by. It is not for his followers to seek the dark causes of war and poverty, or the complicated reasons for their own unfortunate position. He gives them a simple answer for all to say aloud confidently: Who causes war? The Aztecs! Who causes poverty? The Aztecs! Who causes them to lose their pitiful jobs? The Aztecs! Who devised the devilish laws of nature? The Aztecs! With such a simple catechism, it is no wonder he wants to kill off all the intelligent people as fast as he can before they can ask any questions about such a silly way of looking at things.
>
> (p. 3)

So, blame and projection provide one opportunity to locate the cause of threat, misery, and anger outside of oneself, outside of one's collective. This is a dynamic that makes deception appealing. Berne is writing about a form of exploitation. Power can be taken by exploiting the vulnerabilities and fears of the people. To be fearful with anger helps to make an oppressor believable and the oppressed vulnerable to practical and psychological subjugation. As Berne stated, political leanings can be governed by feelings that are raw, rather than by well processed, regulated minds.

Within the theoretical body of Transactional Analysis is a model named symbiosis (Schiff & Lee Schiff, 1971). The original model aimed to capture the decommissioning of some mental functioning through interpersonal dynamics and states of dependency. In other words, the model illustrated natural and pathological dependencies people might have at social, practical, and psychological levels. I am interested in deconstructing some of their work, by placing a radical lens on the intersubjective power dynamics between people. To do that, I will be drawing on political and psychoanalytic concepts.

So far, I have referred to oppression and deception. I have said that it is the deception that allows the subject to open their mind to their oppressor. I borrow from Gramsci (1971/2003) here to describe the unprotected response to an attractive and more powerful other. This leads to the gateway of a process of subjugation in the subject. In Figure 4.2, I draw the ego state model as we know it in TA, depicting the Parent, Adult, and Child. Drawing on the model of symbiosis (Schiff & Lee Schiff, 1971), I illustrate the cathected ego states as solid lines and the decathected states of mind with dotted boundaries. I say more about this as the chapter evolves. The transaction itself I have kept with solid lines as the dynamic is not entirely unconscious. At the social level, there is an agreement between parties for this relationship to happen. This model can be considered at the individual or the collective level.

Collectively speaking, Berne (2020) also noticed the rising role of capitalism and commercial opportunity in the West.

> The average voter has little chance of forming an accurate image of what a candidate is like. He only knows what the candidate and the newspapers tell him, and they both have their axes to grind and will present images fashioned accordingly for public consumption.
>
> (Berne, 2020, p. 1)

Capitalist economic structures and processes provide tremendous opportunity for self-promotion which can be captivating even if based on deception. There is opportunity for communication in abundance in recent decades with the increasing role of social media in our lives. Whilst captivating deception goes back centuries, the power back then was not the capacity of social media, but guns. Guns had been the coveted possessions that had made the slave trade possible. The existing rivalries amongst African tribes could be exploited by Europeans and was so for centuries. This brought the collusion of the slave traders, who "sold out to the merchant ships" (Marley, 1980) largely across the west coast of Africa. Through violence, force, as well as infectious diseases such as smallpox, European troops weakened the African people, fought over their

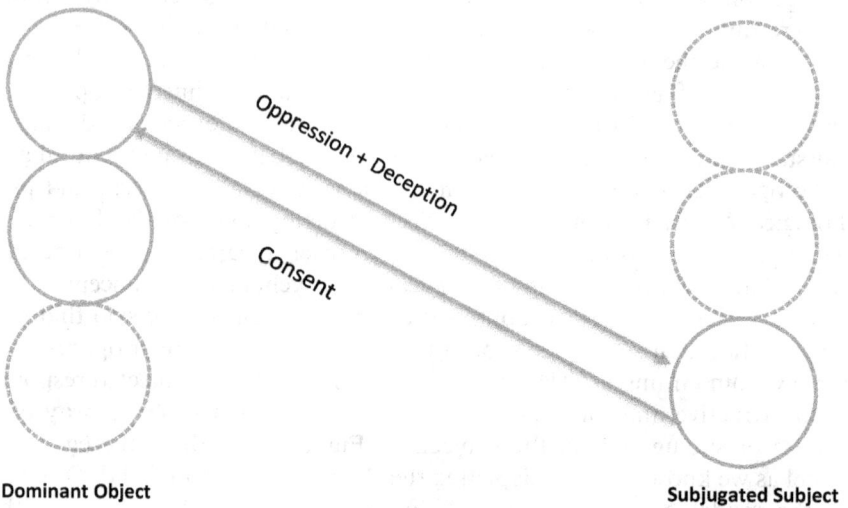

Dominant Object   **Subjugated Subject**

Figure 4.2 Oppression, deception, and consent. Illustration by the author.

lands and resources, and claimed imperial possession. Rivalry for power and resources was the drive for domination alongside the fear that European rivals and neighbours might get more of the share. Driven by a threat of missing out, the Europeans had both competition and a sense of entitlement to facilitate their moves. Their mindset around possession, greed, and the threat of missing out was embodied in an alien way to an African people who lived with the land and a community mindset. Not that rivalry was alien to them—this had after all facilitated a wish for weapons amongst the slave merchants. However, without comprehension of national boundaries, the land as possession, they could not prepare for what the Europeans had in mind. Even if they could, with the force of weapons against them, they would have stood no chance[1].

We could think of the colonising of Africa as an international game[2] of "take it"! (Tudor, 2008). Here, Tudor describes driver[3] dynamics of the entitled grabbing of what they can when they can. He also describes the other position—the polarity, or as we could think of it in TA, the complementary symbiotic role in the game of the unentitled who, as a coping strategy and to maintain relationship, tolerate, absorb, or offer themselves up to "take" whatever comes their way. Such dynamics manifesting in a game could be played on many levels: internationally, nationally, organisationally, and between individuals. The conditions for this game are that there must be a quest for more power when one party already has the advantage. In other words, this is not a fair fight. The other important element, drawing from Bollas (1987), is that the soon to be oppressed must have no idea what the oppressor is up to. Chinnock and Minikin (2015) linked extractive introjection to the colonising process.

Bollas described the deception of one party (to our mind, the "coloniser"), moving in without the "colonised" realising what is happening. The colonised are thereby robbed of aspects of their thinking capacity, emotional resonance, and/or soulful autonomy. In its place, the oppressor/coloniser leaves his or her desires and disturbances. The loss of thinking and identity was described by Bollas as a "catastrophe, from which there may well be no recovery" (p. 166).

I have started this chapter with the story of Africa because of my connection to Nigeria. My experience of Nigeria and the subsequent African countries I have been to represents something core in my personal history as well as it being a feature of global dynamics. In my way of thinking, all history is relevant because we have become a global nation. The interdependence across the world continues and shapes some fundamental ways in which we think, what we expect in our lives, and how we will conduct ourselves. The experience of Africa is relevant to international and national race relations today. It has shaped all of us.

Personal Anecdote

For many years, I owned an allotment[4]. I loved being part of this allotment and having my "plot". It was a place for physical hard work, creativity, and to some extent community spirit. My first site was a corner plot nestled close to a line of trees. This suited me. It was out of the way, more private, and I could get on without too much interference from my neighbours. Or so I thought. Most (but importantly, not all) of the people on the allotment were White, working-class retired men. Their curiosity had been aroused by me joining this group as to what this slight, South Asian looking woman was going to get up to. I daresay they did not hold out much hope for me, and during my first year there, I was subject to a great deal of scrutiny from them. Often, shortly after my arrival, a few of them would troop up to my plot and watch what I was up to. I have memories of them leaning on their spades, shaking their heads often accompanied by sharp intakes of breath. These were offered up as informed warnings intended no doubt for my benefit, such as the danger of putting potatoes in the ground in March before the frost is done. My general inclination in life is to be socially pleasant, so I did my best to humour them, protect myself, and just get on with it. By the end of my first year, I had earned the position of being tolerated, perhaps as a local novelty and, by and large, I was then left in peace.

Much as I liked being near the trees, they compromised my harvest and a few years later, I had the chance to take a second plot which was situated right in the middle of the allotment. This was an open, sunny site with plenty of productive potential. However, I was relentlessly visible there, which as the reader may gather was by and large considered a disadvantage by me. The sun beckoned though, so I took my chance. The unforeseen compensation was that I got to know more of the women who were in the minority and so we developed a little sisterly support for each other. Then there was the lead-up to the Brexit vote in the UK.

The Cameron government had come into power in 2010 and the focus of their policy was austerity, which meant cuts in public spending. Simultaneously, there was the Syrian refugee crisis which was in its sixth year in 2016. Millions of Syrian people were displaced, some of whom were fleeing to Europe. In the UK and other European countries, the threat of hardship was hitting some communities. So this, along with the needs of the migrants, provided opportunity for some sharp swings to right-wing politics. These politicians, supported by the right-wing press, were expressing increasingly hostile views about immigration in general. The written reporting was shocking to me, and I became increasingly concerned about the polarising of views, blatant racism, and the rise in populism that had been legitimised. David Cameron, our prime minister at the time, thought perhaps he could manage this and had taken a reckless decision in my view in inviting a referendum on our EU membership. This polarised positions around immigration further, and we saw demonstrations that were reminiscent of earlier decades—debates on the television seemed little more than "bun fights"[5]. There seemed to be no mentalising, reflection, or informed debate that could take the nation through a meaningful discussion to a more grounded position. It was, in my experience, an exposure to systemic oppression and deception that was alienating me from my country.

My allotment had been my "refuge" and place of restoration until the Brexit epidemic arrived. One of the ring leaders (I will call him Rick) turned on me. As I came through the gates one day, he shouted at the top of his voice, "OH! Here come the immigrants!". I was angry and did the only thing a woman can do in that scenario—summon up some dignity and march with determined resolution to my plot. I daresay my digging was extra deep and ferocious that day. The following week, I had a visit from Rick who launched into a monologue of how "Boris" was going to sort us out. I couldn't help myself and responded with my argument about the devastating consequences leaving the EU would have on our economy and our people. Perhaps he was not used to people answering him back, as it seemed to stop him in his tracks and he said, "do you really think so?". I affirmed and said I hoped that would be enough for us to agree to disagree. Not so. There seemed to be a need in Rick to pay me a visit every time I went down to my plot. Time and time again, I was subjected to his opinions about immigration, the EU, and the need for us as a country to be "sorted out". One day, I wanted to just put a stop to it all. It had become personal, an attack on everything I stood for—my race, my gender, and my views. So, I said something along the lines of, "Rick, I think it best if you and I don't discuss politics". Perhaps he felt rebuffed, though I got a little more space after that. Then, the first time I visited after the Brexit vote, Rick was in an animated circle talking with five or six people. As I came in, he led the jeers and catcalling. Jubilant and triumphant in their victory, I trudged up to my plot, determined not to be pushed out of what I loved doing, but feeling very alone, nonetheless.

As mentioned earlier, systemic deception exploits the threat, fear, and hatred that we are all capable of feeling. During the lead up to Brexit, many people had suffered from the cutbacks and one of the lies told during the campaign was that all of the money spent on the EU could be fed into our National Health System. So, heightening primitive feelings via the imagery of immigrants blocking our health service and false reporting in general was colonising public platforms. "Fake news" with some grains of truth flourished. The compassion for refugees was attacked to such an extent that it ran out in many quarters. It was not just political refugees—economic migrants, especially Black ones from sub-Saharan Africa, were depicted as the enemy—almost as criminals. At times, I felt I was returning to a nightmare—the kind of which I had not known or lived with in full capacity since childhood.

Case Example: Emma

Like Rick, Emma's father was prone to racism. Emma presents a social self that is kind, generous, and open minded. She knows her father was extremely racist and that with enough provocation, she too can resort to a racist state of mind. She feels ashamed of this in herself, and it has been painful to confess this to me. She described the terrible conflict she faced as a child when her father refused to allow her best friend (who was Black) to visit her home. In other words, Emma knows part of her script involves her guilt and sense of "Bad Me" (Sullivan, 1953), for choosing a Black friend. This identity holds when she is with her White family. With me, she experiences some shame, a *Bad Me* that is also connected to feelings of betrayal. In other words, her confusion and challenge with her personal and social scripting is how can she move between a White-excluding environment into one that allows for cross-racial connection? Both experiences involve guilt associated with betrayal to her family, or shame with her chosen companion and therapist for her heritage of White racism. I suggest Emma suppresses these feelings, and they form part of the *Bad Me* identities she wants to forget about. At the same time, there was a deeper split within herself concerning the experiences she had to dissociate from, feelings that she wished to banish, because they represented something other, something that could not be imagined as belonging to her. In other words, "Not Me" (Sullivan, 1953). Her double bind was that there was something fundamentally wrong with her and that in facing her "Bad Me" dilemma, both positions confirmed this. Either abandon your friend and your father may bestow "OKness" or abandon your father and keep your friend, as well as your disloyalty to your family. I understand this bind she was in as a deception. She was conflicted on both counts by a false belief and her feelings of shame and guilt were evoked within because of what she picked up from her family and society.

Understanding oppression accompanied by deception clarifies why political and psychological resistance is so crucial if a person or a people are to retain their soul. It also explains why such courage is not always common. Steve Biko and others paid with their lives for such resistance, while survivors are left traumatised with many complexities added to their scripts.

Script as Double Agent

I think of script[6] (Berne, 1975) as protecting alienated parts of the self from further damage. Simultaneously, by keeping these parts at bay, script contributes to the recesses of our soul. So, the scripting process is simultaneously creative as well destructive. Script protects what can be salvaged yet acts as a kind of double agent because it buys into what is on offer to maintain relationship and connection with community. It is the dialogue an individual creates within an oppressive system. So, in the case of the African people, they were compelled to do business with the Europeans or to die. They had to buy into the new social, political, and economic system that was being thrust upon them and in so doing, the process of cultural alienation began. This was now at risk of being lost, never to be recovered. I argue (Minikin, 2018) that some of these lost components are ejected outside of the script system—they are killed off, dissociated from.

What I describe as a cultural trauma has its parallels in the psychological process of relational trauma. Given the need to survive, identification with the oppressor is key. Ultimately, through forced oppression, there is a requirement for the oppressed to oppress themselves. The less powerful are compelled to identify with the powerful, as we see in the case of Emma. Without that, resistance will continue, causing trouble for the oppressor (Seelye, 2020). Such resistance is possible when certain criteria have been met and I say more about that in the second half of the book. For now, I continue to think about how such deception continues along with the traumatic effect.

Often, people who attend psychotherapy have turned inward, their internalised tyranny killing off aspects of their humanity that have been subjugated. In short, I understand deception as a deep lie on the part of the oppressor, who is determined not to lose a powerful grip on the oppressed. The meaning I make is that aspects of the soul in both the oppressor and the oppressed are killed off or go so far into retreat that recall and recovery is very hard. My fellow gardener at the allotment, Rick, had felt threatened by the images of refugees coming to the UK. He read the newspapers validating and encouraging his fear and his outrage that he will be robbed. This validated his aggression, which was like the kind of hatred and aggression expressed by Emma's father. Subsequently, the goal is to export the feeling of trauma into the vulnerable other—the less powerful. The internalised oppressor lived on inside Emma, traumatising her, terrifying her. It was there because her father could not process his fear, and the same was true of Rick. Fear for some means to be vulnerable and so it is killed off.

Another contemporary writer who describes this well is Daniel Shaw (2014) in his writing about the process of subjugation in traumatising narcissism. He drew from his experience of cults, which may include intergenerational trauma (Minikin, 2011; Noriega, 2010), including the need for the tyrant to find a relational home for his or her disturbance. So, the other is colonised, and the relational dynamic psychologically structured (Little, 2006) and set. Through a colonising process, the oppressed serve to accommodate the badness for the oppressor, with whom the oppressed identify. This means relinquishing some aspect of their selfhood. The relinquishing has come about because of the pacification of their life force. This is represented in Figures 4.2 and 4.3 by the ego states with the dotted lines. In my version of the diagrams, the dotted lines represent the giving up of life force as the giving in to oppression which takes place. This comes about in situations when subjugation facilitates survival. What has been missing in the narrative within Transactional Analysis is the description of power dynamics and the processes of extracting resources from the less powerful other. I look further into this by linking the process of pacification with Bollas ideas on extractive introjection.

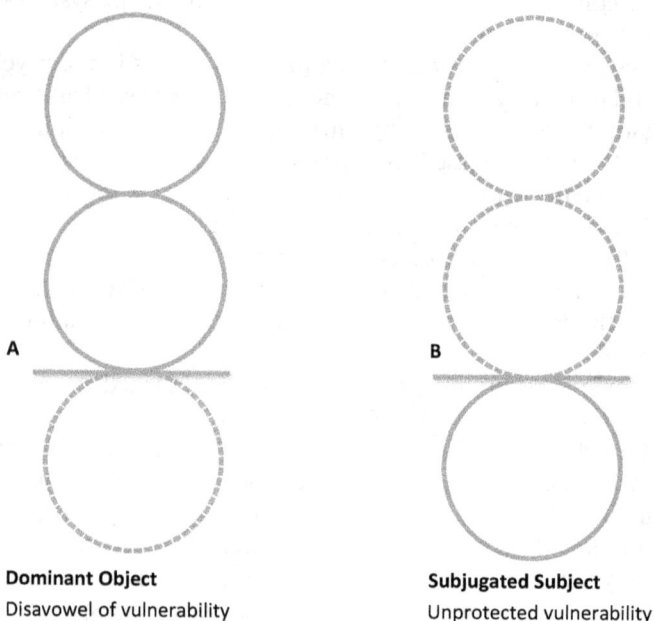

Dominant Object
Disavowel of vulnerability

Subjugated Subject
Unprotected vulnerability

Figure 4.3 Defences against vulnerability. Illustration by the author.

Pacification: Extractive Introjection

Bollas (1987) described that when a subject is robbed of their resources, it is an "intersubjective violence" (p. 158):

> The loss of a part of the self means not only a loss of content, function, and process, but also a loss of one's sense of one's own person. A loss of this nature constitutes a deconstruction of one's history: the loss of one's personal history is a catastrophe, from which there may well be no recovery.
>
> (Bollas, 1987, p. 166)

Figures 4.2 and 4.3 illustrate how resources from the other are consciously or unconsciously taken. They may be skills, knowledge, thinking capacity, emotions, or as described, deep aspects of the self. As a result, the subject is left diminished; hence, the ego states of Parent and Adult are drawn with dotted lines. The taking process is conscious, as it was during colonial times, and it may also be unconscious when aggression or envy is an unknown feature of the object's mind. There is also an unconscious dynamic regarding the transfer of disturbances into the subject's mind. This could include their desires, hatred, sadism, or other disturbances which are then adopted. So, as Bollas describes so well, something is taken and something gets left behind. Traditionally in TA, introjection has been considered as an internalising of the other through the Parent ego state. This is a natural process in relationship though what I am pointing to here, with Bollas' help, is something much more traumatic, something devastating.

Bollas referred to the loss of identity and the sense of self that comes from having a place in the community, society, and culture. His ideas emphasise that it is important to feel rooted historically and environmentally and that to have consciousness about that facilitates an experience of feeling connected. Having security about who you are and who you belong to is diametrically opposed to a sense of alienation. The form of extractive introjection I am referring to here describes the theft of a people's culture and sense of self of the sort that I am describing in relation to Africa.

Returning for a moment to *Things Fall Apart* (Achebe, 1958), the author concludes his novel with a description of the process in the mind of the British Commissioner in Nigeria. The Commissioner finds himself having to deal with the aftermath of a tragedy, whereby the hero of the book, a celebrated Igbo man becomes diminished in his life and ends it with suicide. This of course was representative of what Achebe saw happening to his culture. The book ends with the Commissioner having to deal with the dead man. Contemplating this, he thinks about how he could write about this in the book he was planning. Achebe makes use of irony as he described the Commissioner having an internal dialogue about the book he was planning to write about the domination and submission of the tribes living in the Lower Niger. The Commissioner was wondering how much space in his book he could give to the man that killed himself. Bit by bit, he reduced the space down to one paragraph—a parallel process of the loss of land to the people who had lived there who were now being subjugated and diminished.

Here, Achebe establishes what has been done to his people. He shows that he sees the European mind as it was then. He saw how his people were seen by them. Achebe understood that colonialism was more than a political arrangement. It was an occupation of land, resources, and culture. To extract one culture and impose the superiority of another requires something profound to happen in the minds of the people. Actual political colonialism has clarified something more about this process. Additionally, the role of extractive introjection in the transferential relationship (Chinnock & Minikin, 2015) helps explain something important. Counselling and psychotherapy have been sensitive to supporting the autonomy of clients, though something has very much been missing about the use of authority and the depths of vulnerability in all of us, particularly when we are in a crisis and reaching out for help. Extractive introjection helps to flesh out

51

dynamics of oppression with deception by adding the dimension of theft and loss. It helps account for the decathecting of resources and psychic life. Thus, the diminishing of vitality. As with Emma, her father was dominant in the state of her mind when she came to me. Emma was pacified and "played dead" to diminish his onslaught. This helps intensify the pacification process —and it was necessary because of her dependency on him.

Dependency

> He gives them an image of the world and he gives them a sureness about this image, and sureness is what they want above all. Once they accept this image they act in accordance with it, even in the face of all reality to the contrary.
>
> (Berne, 2020, p. 4)

From the beginning of life, we experience power dynamics through dependency. Even if we consider an individual parent and baby, the parent holds more resources and therefore more power than the baby. Their love for their baby evokes a desire to be responsive, possibly attentive to the infant's subjectivity. Their capacity to do this will have a context depending on how safe, supported, and emotionally literate that parent is. The baby also has some influence and can make demands on the parent through, for instance, crying. This will also have a context depending on the environment and how well the baby is consequently. At times, the unprocessed dynamics in society, as well as within individuals, will be embodied, and there will be limits to responsiveness. So, the baby learns what is and is not possible and what response is most likely to elicit care. I am describing the ingredients that form the basis of socialising, of script, which continues to develop throughout life and is fundamentally designed to facilitate our survival, our belonging, and to keep important people in the here and now in relationship with us. The ordinary dependency that a baby has means, to my mind, that we are all hardwired to engage with and respond most to those whom we see as important, and we are pulled to keep their interest and their care.

I take this human capacity for dependency further to think about how this works in situations that are oppressive rather than responsive. Earlier in this chapter, I drew on ideas about *spontaneous consent* (Gramsci, 1971/2003). The less powerful subject will consent to oppression because there is an economic, social, and/or psychological dependency on the more powerful other. Dependency evokes the experience of options being limited. This diminishes a sense of vitality because there is a genuine as well as a perceived limit to the influence that the subject has. This is potentially a social and economic reality, such as the unemployed being dependent on social benefits to make ends meet. This not only affects their resources, but it also affects their negotiating capacities in social and political forums and elevates their experience of dependency. If they are lucky, politicians might fight their corners for them. Thus, they depend on others who are closer to the centre who may offer or withhold. Gramsci's ideas explain how the division of power means the mind of the oppressed is controlled in a way that is like scripting, whereby an infant learns to consent to his or her caregivers. Their vulnerability in this situation is not known to them, because as Bollas cites, the subject needs to have no idea what the object is up to while complying. So, when there is an alienating relational dynamic, the oppressor needs to disavow their vulnerability whilst the oppressed are unconscious to the necessity for protection. The three dynamics necessary in my view for oppression to be sustained are deception, dependency and pacification. Relationally speaking, they are facilitated by extractive introjection and a disavowal of vulnerability in the oppressor.

Returning to Emma

It seemed impossible for Emma to find her protesting voice. For multiple reasons, her father was traumatised. Part of his trauma was the risk of death due to a medical condition hanging over him throughout Emma's child-hood. He raised Emma alone, so she was utterly dependent on him. Her compulsion to maintain relationship was necessary. Her potential outrage at her father's tyranny was too threatening for their bond, so she killed it off. The extent and depth of this process could not be reached through words. Many months into our work, I became infected with an overwhelming drag into sleep. No amount of caffeine, sugar, fresh air, rosemary, or peppermint oil could keep me awake. I was infused with a leaden, incapacitating deadening of mind and body. Session after session I would droop. In con-trast, Emma would chat her way through my slumbers, seemingly unaware of my state. Understanding from supervision pointed to unconscious rage.

This invited me to consider projective identification (Ogden, 1979) and dissociation in my countertransference. However, cognitive insight alone seemed unable to help. I could understand our dynamic in terms of an en-actment (Stern, 2011), whereby I was manifesting the deadness in Emma that I could psychically identify with. Aspects of her liveliness had been under profound psychic attack, and this was something I could relate to. At this point there was the danger that my capacity for engagement with Emma was so shut down that the therapy between us would be "killed off". Thinking further about how vitality between us was being obliterated, I recognised that both of us had a complex relationship with protest. We experienced this as threatening to a critical bond, and hence this evoked a "Not Me" state.

"Not Me" encounters in society are expressed in the narrative of totalitarian politics that champion forceful power over anything threatening or hated. This validates intolerance, hatred, and tyrannical states of minds in citizens. Dealing with difference in this way promotes banishing and death which rids the State of possible relatedness with that "Other". Psychically and politically, these oppressive dynamics, as part of alienation seek satisfaction through vengeance. I return to my work with Emma in the second part of the book (in chapter nine) where I consider further the dynamics of trauma, dissociation and enactments.

I have argued here that compliance to oppressive systems is possible because of the dynamics of deception, pacification, and dependency. These processes are the subconscious dynamics that maintain oppressive economic, social, and psychological systems. I have indicated in this chapter that these experiences are traumatic—they are death dealing. The following two chapters include conversations between myself and two of my colleagues. They continue the theme of trauma and consider the intergenerational and transgenerational trauma that comes collectively and directly through our ancestral lines.

Postscript

Looking at a map of pre-colonial Africa, we see that the territories are fluid, and some tribes such as the Fulani and Masai moved with the seasonal changes. Partly owing to the slave trade, the continent was not heavily populated, and the resources were rich not only in gold, but also in coffee and chocolate that the Europeans had gained a taste for.

> The Scramble for Africa, also called the Partition of Africa, Conquest of Africa, or the Rape of Africa, was the invasion, occupation, division, and colonization of African territory by European powers during a short period known to historians as the New Imperialism (between 1881 and 1914). The 10 percent of Africa that was under formal European control in 1870 increased to almost 90 percent by 1914, with only Ethiopia (Abyssinia) and Liberia remaining independent. European motives included the desire to control valuable natural resources, rivalry and the quest for national prestige, and religious missionary zeal. Internal African politics also played a role.

> The Berlin Conference of 1884, which regulated European colonization and trade in Africa, is usually referred to as the starting point of the Scramble for Africa. There were considerable political and economic rivalries among the European empires in the last quarter of the 19th century. Partitioning Africa was effected largely without Europeans going to war. In the later years of the 19th century, the European nations transitioned from "informal imperialism"—i.e., exercising military influence and economic dominance—to direct rule, bringing about colonial imperialism.
>
> (Wikipedia, 2023, paras. 1–2)

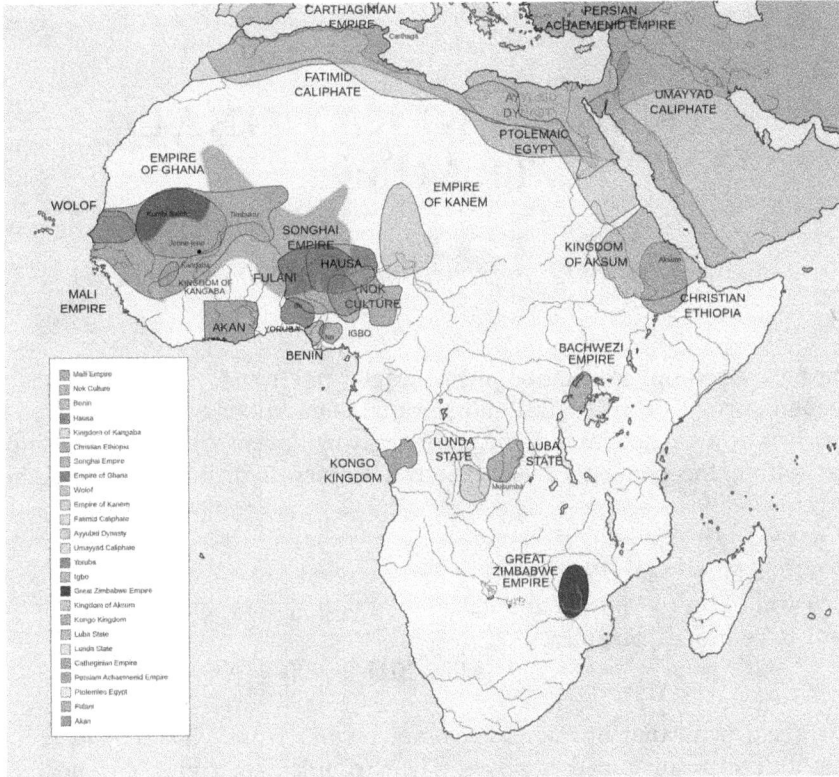

Figure 4.4 Map of pre-colonial African civilisations. (Image by Jeff Israel, 2007, reproduced from Wikimedia Commons under CC BY-SA 3.0.)

Source: https://commons.wikimedia.org/w/index.php?curid=2660560

Notes

1 See map of pre-colonial Africa, fig 4.4
2 In TA, a game describes the dynamics between individuals, groups, or institutions that can lead to defensive or destructive outcomes.
3 In TA, drivers describe the defensive behaviours, or "winning formulas" that people learn to manage relationships and life.
4 An allotment in the UK is a rented piece of land shared amongst the local community. It is divided into individual plots and is made available to grow vegetables, flowers, and/or fruit.
5 This is an English metaphor sometimes used to depict an argument based on petty views that do not develop or inform important issues.
6 "Script" in Transactional Analysis is the unconscious narrative created within a mind, in response to relational and social experiences. Script drives the expectations and dramas that people live out.

5

TRANSGENERATIONAL
TRAUMA

(with contributions from Dharmacharini Jayakara)

During a week-long meditation, my colleague and friend, Eugene Ellis, made some important psychological and spiritual connections with his father. He describes how connecting with his father only made sense if he could position that within the context of his ancestral history that shaped both father and son:

> After many years of unlocking the unsayable;
> I want you to know that I have heard you,
> I have heard your plea.
>
> (Ellis, 2021, p. 88)

It is a sad truth that our parents cannot save us from what they have not been able to resolve in themselves. Their troubles, their anxiety, and their trauma is inflicted upon our undefended selves and if they haven't been able to make sense of it themselves, what can we do about it? So, we learn how to make the best of things via our scripts, and we absorb unprocessed trauma including what I have been referring to as "unformulated experiences" (Stern, 2011) into our bodies and they help constitute our most fundamental reactions to what life presents.

Whilst we have conscious experience of our parents, memories of the ways in which we felt injured by them, the transmission of unformulated experiences from our ancestors may feel more nebulous, as is the transmission of trauma from the collective. Transgenerational trauma is an enigmatic feature that may seem somewhat incredulous to a rational mindset, yet to a radical mind, it needs exploration, examination, and deconstructing within our contemporary ways of living and communicating. Without such thought, we are in danger of abstaining and witnessing the ongoing rise in populism (see Lewis, 2019). I say this given social media's escalating capacity to run all sorts of political and social campaigns, based on the premise of advertising. Some of these communicate bigotry, prejudice, and opinions deliberately intending to exploit fear, harbour hatred, and communicate messages based on opinions rather than understanding. These are now of far-reaching and

DOI: 10.4324/9780429289231-6

global proportions and can have devastating impacts. Whilst I would argue a case for Demelza Frazier's[1] achievement, in equal measure I feel concerned of the potential of social media to reach such vast audiences so quickly in a way that leaves us all vulnerable to not being given time and capacity to be informed, or to reflect, consider, and talk meaningfully with each other about important matters. Our global economy binds us to international structures and processes, and I would argue that it is these that may eventually destroy our planet. We find it hard to give up what we have for the greater good.

I propose unprocessed emotional and traumatic material is passed on from one generation to the next and across the collective, manifesting in embodied ways through our economic, social, and political structures, as well as within our individual bodies. It is hard to grasp how the impact of history lives on and how it can be embellished in contemporary times. Whilst progress in some areas has been achieved, it seems easy to swing back and close down in older more parochial mindsets as soon as trouble stirs.

This chapter and the next are based on a discussion between two women. In this chapter, I illustrate how and why slavery is relevant to all of us—not just Black people. Using insight from colonialism and slavery, I consider the legacy that these two long-term historical events bring. I make use of my own personal and professional experience to illustrate the challenges in being aware of and working with transgenerational trauma. My personal interests are with slavery, colonialism, and indenture and my reading on these topics has been drawn from writers interested in transgenerational trauma. For those living away from Africa, yet with ancestral connections to the continent—especially West Africa—the recovery from the violating trauma of slavery remains ongoing work. For the rest of us, we are implicated historically and in ongoing life in all sorts of ways.

Conference Example

For many years now, I have attended an annual (BAATN) conference in the UK that is for Asian, African, Caribbean, and multi-heritage therapists. One year the speaker was a Black woman from the Caribbean who spoke with great vitality and humour about her experiences in an academic teaching department. Her talk was robust, informative, and captivating. Afterwards, I approached her as I wanted to congratulate her. As I started my enthusiastic appreciation, her eyes deadened, dropped to the ground, and she murmured a thank you. I felt lost, confused at the loss of vitality between us. We joined the queue for lunch, took our food, and the only seats free were two together. So, we sat, making polite remarks about the tastiness of the food, when a friend burst in on us. "Oi! Karen!" My friend rushed to me, and I stood so we could greet each other with a hug. No sooner had she pulled her chair to join us, another friend joined in. They were both Black and as we started our animated talk, all four of us came to life. In our group of four, where there has been mutual knowing and history, we could all start enjoying each other and start the job of building bridges of connection amongst strangers. Because that is what I had encountered earlier—an experience of feeling estranged from someone I wished to know more.

It wasn't till I left the conference and walked to the train station that I got it. The speaker had seen me as White. My Whiteness had been the encounter for both of us. It was a crucial moment for me. I had to face up to my part-Whiteness and recognise what that may have meant. My embodiment of Whiteness has afforded me relative privileges in life, and it had been a barrier to connection with my new Black colleague. When I recounted the story to some White colleagues in later years, who would see me as a racial "other", they responded with anger: "She didn't see you!" they claimed as they rushed to my psychological defence and protection. But, of course, she did ... she saw the side of me that is also a part of who I am when I am with Black people. Much as I feel I understand, and as much as I have seen and felt the racist gaze (Keval, 2016) upon me, I have the privilege of protection too. It is well documented that lighter skinned people are not subjected to the same hatred, fear, and intolerance than the darker.

I had witnessed something of the trauma that had been passed down through the generations for hundreds of years and whilst an aspect is specific to Black women, I also needed to check in with my vulnerabilities and demands for relationship. In that moment of her deadening before me, averting her gaze, she showed me the "breaking" of the Black woman. During slavery and beyond, Black women have experienced the most unthinkable degradations, mental and physical torture in attempts to "break" their spirit. This "breaking" of slaves was described by Lynch, reportedly a British slave owner in the West Indies, that came to America to instruct other slave owners about how to keep their slaves under control. Difficult though it is to repeat some words from his speech in Virginia, I offer an example, that illustrates how he, his peers, and the wider White collective understood the significance of alienation in retaining power. In particular they understood how to violate the men in the presence of women, then legitimately rape the women, who would then become their servants in the psychological task of "breaking":

> Keep the body, take the mind! In other words, break the will to resist ... Take the female and run a series of tests on her to see if she will submit to your desires willingly. Test her in every way, because she is the most important factor for good economics. If she shows any sign of resistance in submitting completely to your will, do not hesitate to use the bull whip on her to extract that last bit of resistance out of her. Take care not to kill her, for in doing so, you

spoil good economic. When in complete submission, she will train her off springs in the early years to submit to labor when they become of age.

(Lynch, 1712, p. 29)

The story of Black women descended from slavery points to the complexity of gender politics and intersectionality (Crenshaw, 1989). Just as the women during slavery had witnessed terrible violence, so have other Black women been subjected to terrible physical and mental torture. I argue that slavery set up a mindset about who and what Black men and women were and what White people were entitled to do to them. Slavery paved the way for subsequent imperialism, colonialism, and the political, economic, and cultural domination of Africa by Europeans. One terrible example of individual suffering (there are many) is the treatment of Winnie Mandela during captivity. Nelson Mandela was confined with his colleagues and no doubt humiliated in prison. However, the degradation of Winnie Mandela was on another level. There is much more to say about the dynamics of intersectionality in culture and society, so my brief mention here hardly does the subject justice. Suffice to acknowledge that when those with power fear threat of loss, shocking violating dynamics and actions surface. For Winnie Mandela, there was no end to it all once she was released from prison, as she was banished from her home, her family, and friends—forced to live in an area where she could not speak the local language. Her experiences as a woman, a wife, and a mother are truly shocking to read about and it is a wonder she survived it all—such was her resolve, her determination, her necessary rage. This is not to condone acts of vengeance and killing, but to understand them and to see that in the face of unthinkable horrors people kill or get killed. So, it is within our mind. Our cultural and intergenerational traumas haunt us and intersect with our significant relationships, all of which are internalised, identified with, repressed, and/or dissociated from. It is our dependency on more powerful others who oppress that leaves us vulnerable to killing off vital parts of our being.

I have to push myself and ask why it feels so necessary to write about these experiences in my lifetime? I cannot not answer the question completely or simply, just as I could not explain why Alex Haley's story, "Roots", reached right into me—into my core, as did the music of Bob Marley, Jimmy Cliff, the writings of Toni Morrison, Alice Walker, James Baldwin. I know I have lived close to the Black experience and feel it as if it spoke to a part of me ... and perhaps in ways it has done. But there are missing pieces here and I have to dig deeper or search closer to home somehow. So, following on from my earlier story of the conference, I decided to talk in the here and now with other women. What follows first is a transcript of a "race conversation" (Ellis, 2021) between me and a Black friend and colleague of Jamaican heritage. I had some thoughts prior to it of the sort of areas we could talk about that might reflect experiences of transgenerational trauma. The questions may have served as a trigger, but when we met, we spoke spontaneously. We were two British women listening, linking, and reflecting on themselves.

The Process and Set Up

In order to provide some structure, I sent these questions to Jayakara. The idea was that we would both hold these lightly but use them to trigger some memories, thoughts, and reflections before we spoke.

- We have spent many years at BAATN's (Black, African, and Asian Therapy Network) conferences coming together to reflect on the experiences of being Black or Asian therapists in Britain. What stands out for us as we think of these experiences?
- What has evolved personally and professionally for us in terms of learning?
- How do we think the encounters and conversations have changed over the years?
- Can we remember when we first realised our transgenerational heritage? What was that like for us?
- How does our heritage influence our way of seeing our social and psychological worlds?
- How does our awareness of oppressive systems such as slavery and colonialism influence our work as psychotherapists, supervisors, and trainers? What does it make us sensitive to?
- What do we notice in our clients and students who have these experiences in their history?
- Does this change how we think about ego states and scripts?

This is what we captured:

Jayakara: I feel anxious I won't be able to answer your questions.
Karen: Like you gotta know something?
Jayakara: Yeah, like—who am I? What do I know?

This first question from Jayakara seemed key and we spent some time exploring "who am I?"

Who am I?: Ancestral Callings

Jayakara: I'll tell you where I went to ... questions four and five got me thinking of my ancestry. [Question four: Can we remember when we first realised our transgenerational heritage? What was

60

that like for us? Question five: How does our heritage influence our way of seeing our social and psychological worlds?]

Jayakara: I had always thought that my great grandmother was Asian. I always assumed my great grandfather was from Syria—or Lebanon. And that my Dad's side were from Africa. My mum talked more (about her family) than my dad ... there is the family trauma and then colonial trauma, and it is hard to separate, and you cannot really. I was interested whether my great grandfather or great great grandfather was born in Jamaica. And I started reading about Syrians in Jamaica and they only started coming in 1891 ... from the Lebanese mountains that were in Syria then.

Karen: So ... you wanted to know, to go and find out—what was the journey? What lived experiences did your ancestors have that haven't been talked about? Which *stories are broken ... lost ...*

Jayakara: Yeah ... then I asked my granny's cousin ...*And it just shows ... she did not know [about the family's heritage].* Then I asked my mum's brother and he kept saying "*I don't know—we didn't talk about those things*" [Jayakara's mother is deceased].

I was affected by Jayakara's searching for lost stories, her attempts to piece her history together, to discover how and why her ancestors came to Jamaica. She seems to be holding both the history of the slave trade, a history of cut-off roots and silencing of identity, and destruction of culture. The slaves had their names taken and were renamed—all they were, what they had known—gone. Meanwhile the emigration of the Lebanese and Syrian people to Jamaica at the end of the 19th century happened because they were fleeing persecution from the Ottoman empire. It means that my friend holds the embodiment of fleeing from persecution, capacity to resettle and build a life in a new land, as well as slavery. Further into the conversation, I asked her how she thought her history affected her.

Skin Deep: Internalised Racism and Shadeism

Jayakara: How this affects me? That's confusing ... I've probably told you this story ... I can remember granny talking to mum and saying, "*Him Black you know! ...him Black!*" [Said in a derogatory way]. They were talking about another man who had dark skin. However, my dad is dark. It didn't make sense cos in England we were just a Black family. And yet ...

Karen: You're talking about how "alive" shadeism was ... how alive ... and that is a legacy, isn't it?

Jayakara: Yeah and on the one hand mum was talking about it, then she'd get very upset when people said ... "well you know one of your parents must be White". She didn't like looking like mixed race. She wanted her Jamaican credentials but at the same time she's putting down people for being Black, or really dark, or having "nappy" hair. So, that was confusing.

Karen: The contradictions of her wanting to be seen for who she was, who her people were.

Jayakara: Yup.

Karen: And not be projected onto because she had fair skin.

Jayakara: Yeah she was very proud of being Jamaican. My dad was proud of being Jamaican but also wanted to be English if you know what I mean. Like he was proud that the minister in his parish in Jamaica was a German minister, so almost like, "Yeah he was a German, a really good preacher".

Karen: So, real confusion in identifying with the old coloniser but at the same time ...

Jayakara: Wanting to almost be them.

Karen: It seems like something fragmenting happens and that slices of the story get lost—which is what I thought you were saying to me when you went to the older generation. Like you want to find those pieces and put them back somehow. Your German preacher was reminding me of my time in Nigeria when I was growing up and how some educated Nigerians wanted to lose their Nigerian accent, to speak English with an English accent. So that strange mix of wanting independence (from the colonial power) but at the same time, the system has got them.

This part of the conversation highlights the confusion and contradictions around internalised transgenerational racism. The introjection of the oppression lives on, as does the extraction (Bollas, 1987), the loss of parts of identity. The breaking of the narrative gives opportunity for oppressed selves to live alongside the internalised oppressor. However, the fragments of life, of pride, identity, and culture come up for a breath and do what they can through the wreckage of trauma to build some muscle power with what lives on. So, this life force can co-create, ebb and flow, and "rise" (Angelou, 1986). In this next extract, Jayakara illustrates the humiliation of Black men through this example with her father. This again is key, as we see in the next chapter and as we saw in the case of the Black England football players during the summer of 2021[2].

UK in the 1950s: Lost Stories, Confusion, Humiliation

Jayakara: My father was bought up with his cousins and grandmother. He comes from near Mandeville, but his mum worked in Montego

Bay, for a superintendent—someone who was quite powerful. She was a nanny and then became head housekeeper, and he (my dad) was proud of that. Some of the White people in Jamaica (who visited the superintendent's home and who my dad knew) had said when you come to England, look us up. They lived in Richmond, and so he did go and look them up, and they just shooed him away, "What are you doing here?"

Karen: What is common in my history and yours is something of these lost stories ... In the early 1960s, I walked the streets of London with my father—I don't remember the racist attacks. I was only told recently that they came regularly. But he hasn't talked about it. But perhaps he wanted to pass on some kind of pride to his kids, not shame and the horror, and helplessness—and rejection. The rejection for your father of going and knocking on the door of those English folk and being told to go away!

Jayakara: Yup.

Karen: Its very confusing when you have idealised the country that now people are rejecting you from.

UK in the 1960s–1970s: Progression and Oppression

Jayakara: And that thing of being born in the sixties—like everything was possible ... there were schools, youth clubs, sport.

Karen: A time of optimism.

Jayakara: Yeah, like if your parents didn't have anything it didn't matter cos school provided it ... I can remember starting school with mostly White kids. This is infant school and then by the time I entered junior school it was mostly Black and Asians—or 50/50. There had been a "White flight" from my home area. We moved in and the Whites moved out.

Karen: So, there was movement, people moving in and people moving out ... a feeling of optimism alongside everything ... things beginning to open up yet loads of racism, of rejection ... a time also of liberal growth?

Jayakara: I definitely felt that in the junior school ... and then ... I recounted this the other day—I was in the top class (in secondary school). They did not stream us originally which was wonderful. But when they streamed us, something became obvious. I was the only Black kid in the top class. There were two in second and third stream and the majority where in the bottom stream, the fifth class.

Karen: So, like something happened as soon as the hierarchy was imposed—something got highlighted.

63

Jayakara: Yeah and I still remember my mum coming to the open evening ... and probably for the first time feeling really angry at mum's ignorance ... I mean going along with what the teachers say and even though I was near the top of the class in everything. All subjects, right, but still half of the teachers said I could not do "O" level. ["O" levels were the General Certificate in Education.]

Karen: Bloody hell! What, that you couldn't do "O" level—you had to do CSE [Certificate in Secondary Education—a lesser qualification].

Jayakara: Yeah—and I couldn't understand ...

Karen: ... the logic of that.

Jayakara: No and luckily the only CSE I ended up doing was chemistry cos there wasn't enough girls to do "O" level, so I had to do CSE if I wanted to do chemistry. And I wanted to do physics but there wasn't any physics in our school.

Karen: The sexism too! So, something important about finding your way through the system and having these encounters and confusions. How to have your own mind as a clever teenager.

Jayakara: Yeah so I went to grammar school to do my A levels in the end. And there it was all right if you were "special" or "just one".

Karen: Like the special mascot or something?

Jayakara: Yeah ... and as long as you did well, you were one of them.

Karen: Or tolerated?

Jayakara: Yeah.

The 1960s and 1970s seem to represent many things to Jayakara and myself. The era embodied a sense of consciousness raising where both oppression and progression existed in tension with each other. This outward and global experience mirrors how our minds work. Back and forth, retracting and expanding as trauma and script get a hold, then resistance and fightbacks push forth.

Politics and "Politics"

Karen: So, my mind went back to how your mum has a diverse heritage and history. Her Black identity is very complex. She's part of three or four continents. What you said about your dad was he was largely African descent.

Jayakara: Ok. So, going back to my dad (he was a joiner) and he always read newspapers. So, my mum was personally more pushy but not politically aware. My dad was more politically savvy, and he always watched the 6 pm, 9 pm, and 10 pm news. It was annoying he would always want the TV turned on to the news, whether we liked it or not! So, he really was for Idi Amin in terms of Black people having the land back. Then, I went into the 6th form, there were two guys there from Uganda—so I got ...

Karen: ... conflicted.

Jayakara: Yeah—seeing and knowing they had really suffered. But he (dad) talked about the land, and he really liked Muhammad Ali ...

Karen: Like he could take some pride in Black men—powerful Black men.

Jayakara: Yeah.

Karen: And hungry to see the role models of the boldness and fighting spirit in them. It must have been quite radical at the time to hear Muhammad Ali talk—because we hadn't seen much of that before.

Jayakara: Yeah, yeah.

Karen: Those early days of Black consciousness were very powerful. They were very powerful for me, let alone Black men.

As Jayakara was talking, memories of powerful Black men were emerging in my mind. I too remembered the excitement of Muhammad Ali talking and taking on White normative frames of reference. He challenged them at the time, in a different way from another Black hero, "James Baldwin". Both eloquent and bold, and powerful. It was enormously inspirational for me and served to open up spaces in a fresh way in both the US and the UK.

Going Back—Re-Imagining the Eras

Karen: And your dad ... when was he born—in the 1930s?

Jayakara: 1926, and mum was 1939.

Karen: So, when he was born ... in the 1920s and that time, there was conformity and pressure to be good ... It would have been hard to dream that anyone like Muhammad Ali or Idi Amin could have happened—must have been so radical for him ...

Jayakara: Mum—she used to like those radical singers—Bill Withers and Otis Redding ... if you listen to those political songs ... and she had American friends in the army. One friend went to Vietnam and came back traumatised.

Karen: Well ... her world view ... came in more subconsciously with the music and atmosphere in the house ...

Jayakara: Yeah, I picked that up—what they were singing about. And the Americans with their civil rights ... I had a naïve view that

Black Americans had a good life. But the reality was not that and isn't that at all.

Karen: And we are born of that era you and I. So ... how do these fragments come through in our here and now lives? How do these lost stories affect us? How are they still lived but not consciously? Because we can only live with what is conscious like you've been doing—building the story. But how to capture that which hasn't been spoken about but is known somehow within us?

Jayakara: What has come to my mind is something I did with my Buddhist women group. We spoke about when we first became aware of (the impact on ourselves of) our race. This is embarrassing but it is true. Like my brothers could go out with White and Black girls, but White boys wouldn't be interested in me. Only Black boys would be interested in me.

Karen: It is really painful for a girl becoming a woman, isn't it? I remember my mum saying things about who would want me ... conveying that feeling of somehow being second rate. So, you felt White boys just wouldn't be interested in you ...

Jayakara: We would all go to youth clubs, and it was nice. A lot of friends and mixed relationships, and I started going to the Marcus Garvey[3] club. So, I felt safer to go out with the Black guys as at least I knew who I was in that. And I had so many difficulties (with family identities and family problems) that I couldn't have coped with also being undermined by a White guy ... Though there was one nice guy, I met on holiday actually ... south of France. I was 20 and we went out and I really liked him ... I wondered if it would just be whilst we were on holiday, but we arranged to meet up back home. And we met up and he came (travelled 90 miles) and said he wanted to tell me in person that he was back together with his ex-girlfriend. He said he didn't want to just write or phone, he wanted to meet me and tell me. He was a nice guy, and I would have continued to see him ...

Karen: A vulnerable making time ...

Jayakara: Yeah and yet ... my son's 18th birthday party, about 18 people came from those he has gone to college with ... White kids and Black kids ... White boys going out with Black girls, Black boys going out with White girls, Indian and Chinese youngsters all together—so lovely ... and I thought how things have changed ...

Karen: Like there is an ease ... whereas in our day there was awkwardness ...

Jayakara: Felt like they just saw who they wanted to ... I still like it when I walk down the street and I like seeing a Black girl with a White guy.

Karen: One of my best friends at school—a White girl … Her father was a vicar in Balsall Heath[4]. In his church, everyone was West Indian, and her brother went out with a girl from Antigua … Then when I came down south as an adult there just weren't Black or Asian folks around. But in Nigeria there were a lot of mixed families, especially at the university—Black men married to White women and White men with Nigerian women …

Jayakara: That grounding stands you in good stead.

Karen: Maybe something like that …

Reflections

This ends the first of two talks with another woman, a friend, and a colleague. This recapturing of what has happened in our lives, shared experiences, and the struggles of our parents and ancestors is paving the way for part two. How to recover traumas and give them shape, a place, a story? From this conversation, I turn now to another. One that brings together two daughters both of whom hold the partition of India in their histories. I now move on to a conversation between myself and Farah Cottier, a colleague and friend who shares a similar heritage to myself.

Notes

1 This was the 17-year-old girl who filmed George Floyd's murder. She was awarded the Pulitzer prize in 2021.
2 I refer to the abuse inflicted on the Black players who missed the penalty shootout in the final of Euro 2020.
3 Marcus Garvey was a Jamaican political activist.
4 A part of Birmingham where many Black and Asian families live.

6

PARTITION AND INTERGENERATIONAL HAUNTINGS

(with contributions from Farah Cottier)

Daddy, this is our legacy.
But what of us; playing our part in this dance from the past.
With no balm to soothe the corners of the mind,
Which lock away that loveless dread.
That, which is our inheritance.

(Ellis, 2021, p. 88)

Conflict is a necessary factor of society and the problem consists in its proper institutionalisation and canalisation, or if one prefers the psychoanalytical idiom, sublimation.

(Hussain, 1966, p. 33)

At the time of reviewing this chapter, there were approximately 23 countries in the world that were at war, and 14 of those were in Africa. The UK government had just released plans intending to send all single adults that are asylum seekers crossing the channel to Rwanda. Rwanda is to be paid £120 million per year for the next five years to accommodate them. It is a one-way ticket. To live in an atmosphere of war or any kind of armed conflict is to live in an atmosphere of splitting, of totalitarian states of mind, and it is to encounter deep-seated terror based also on witnessing terrible, horrific sights and knowing that inhumane acts are happening around you. As a child, this experience left me feeling profoundly unsafe in my skin. In the West we have seen this in many countries via our screens and we are being faced with such experiences closer to home as we witness today what is happening between Russia and Ukraine. In this chapter, we (Farah and Karen) recollect the encounter with partition experienced by our fathers.

This is the second of two conversations considering the meaning of lost stories with transgenerational trauma. Here, the sense of intergenerational hauntings (Novak, 2022) emerges as two women share their reflections on

DOI: 10.4324/9780429289231-7

how context, conflict, colonialism, and the partition of India contributed to our fathers' identity and capacity to make a life for themselves as immigrants[1]. We think about what was spoken, what was shared, and what was withheld by way of piecing together commonalities in our stories. Our connections and disconnections with our fathers' experiences are efforts to make some sense of our experience and heritage. This theme continues in similar and different ways from part one where we (Karen and Jayakara) reflected on what has not been spoken of. The lost stories and fragmented narratives are recounted as I and Farah aim to make some meaning of experiences of shame, pride, abuse, and trauma from the people who lived before.

Untold Stories: Partition

The year 2020 marked the centenary for the end of indenture, a system of bonded labour that was instituted following the abolition of slavery. The year also marked the 50th anniversary of a new beginning: Fijian Independence. Following the abolition of slavery in the 19th century, a new system of labour was introduced. Indentured labour first appeared on the Indian Ocean islands of Reunion and Mauritius in the 1830s, eventually resulting in 2 million young Indians being transported across the world.

Until recently, the end of colonialism, marked by the partition of India, was an untold story for me (Karen) in the UK. With the 70th anniversary in 2017, TV documentaries such as "My Family, Partition and Me" (Burley, 2017a, 2017b), radio programmes such as "Partition" (Gallagher et al., 2017a, 2017b, 2017c), and a British-made film, "Viceroy's House" (Berges et al., 2017), have enabled personal and regional stories about partition to surface and capture the minds and imaginations of many people in the UK[2]. For some, it has felt like an opportunity to claim an unknown heritage. For me, my colleague and friend, Farah Cottier, partition has been one of the missing pieces from our legacy. We both have fathers who were raised in colonial India and who witnessed partition as young men, before subsequently migrating to Europe for further education and a better life. Like so many others of their generation, our fathers found it difficult to talk about what they saw and experienced during partition. Both had experience of migration within India, Pakistan, and then to Europe. These experiences included traumas, atrocities, and losses. In Europe, there was a need to adjust to a new culture, landscapes, climate, and people amidst the explicit racism, hatred, and discrimination of the 1960s and 1970s. These later social, political, and psychological processes of alienation (Steiner et al., 1975) added to those previously encountered in colonial India and during its subsequent partition.

This section written by myself and Farah continues with the personal and professional contemplations as before. We share the psychological impact of colonialism and the political and social traumas inherent from our perspectives. We consider some of the ways in which these traumas made an impact consciously and unconsciously on our fathers and subsequently on us. Throughout our narrative, we make links between the personal and the political.

We start by considering the history and the legacy of colonialism before its violent end in India. Picking up on the links between political history and psychology, we think about the political and psychological impact of partition and its aftermath. We wonder about the lack of processing around loss, a crisis in belonging and identity. We consider how this legacy has made its impression on us, as daughters, and how we approach our clinical work.

Contemporary Perspectives on Colonialism

Reflecting now, in this postmodern, postcolonial world, it can still feel shocking to recount the arrogance of colonialism and how it was ever possible in the first place. It was, in fact, possible because a number of social, political, and economic conditions were present. As discussed in Chapter Four regarding Africa, the culture and social organisation under colonial rule drew Europeans together because of financial and lifestyle benefits. The capacity to disregard the other—especially people of colour—had long been established through years of slavery. Essentially, the whole notion of White supremacy and imperialism became a driving force during and after slavery because taking control of nations rich in natural resources brought huge economic benefit to the West.

Chinnock and Minikin (2015) argue that there had to be a relational process to make this possible. In other words, the colonisers' wish to move in was not enough—somehow the colonised had to imagine there was some benefit to them—it had to make sense to both parties. As described in the previous chapter, one of the key processes was to create a dependency of the colonised on the coloniser. We have thought of this as a form of political and social symbiosis (Fanon, 1952/2021, p. 64). During and since independency, a wide range of research and writing has described the social and psychological consequences—one seminal text being *Black Skin, White Masks* (Fanon, 1952/2021), in which Fanon describes so powerfully the way in which nations and people were robbed of their identity—their culture, their spiritual beliefs, and connections and society. As their social structures and cultures fell apart, the people were subjugated to the "superiority" of the coloniser:

> Every colonised people—in other words, every people in whose soul an inferiority complex has been created by the death and burial of its local cultural originality—finds itself face to face with the language of the civilising nation.
>
> (Fanon, 1952/2021, p. 9)

This psychological aftermath of colonialism persists in terms of struggles with economies, conflictual politics, and in areas of diaspora, a confusion around identity, and potential loss of pride. All of this making an impact on the cultural sense of self.

In any relationship, including the psychotherapeutic one, people are vulnerable to these powerful intersubjective processes. The subjective loss of aspects of the mind can become unconscious as people become persuaded of the benefits of buying into a new frame of reference. It is on top of these experiences of seduction, exploitation, and mystification that the hurried process of partition took place. We now summarise some of the key events of partition and then follow that with the psychological aftermath that we experienced through our fathers.

Unprocessed Loss: Partition and its Aftermath

The partition of India displaced around 14 million people on religious grounds (see Figure 6.1), and while the number who died has never been clearly confirmed, estimates range between 200,000 and 2,000,000 people (Talbot & Singh, 2009, p. 2). Figure 6.1 illustrates the changing political face of India, Pakistan, and Bangladesh. As previously stated, the lead-up to 1947 was traumatic and many photographs available on the internet document some of the atrocities that were committed. We include links to photographs depicting atrocities at the end of this chapter (see note 20). Accompanying the numerous horrific acts of violence and killings directed against men and boys, there was violence committed against women; around 100,000 women are said to have been kidnapped, raped, humiliated, and/or subjected to slavery (Singh, 2002). Such violations are seemingly a part of the retributive violence and other forms of "ethnic cleansing" that have taken place across the globe throughout history. At the time of writing this, we continue to hear of similar horrors from Myanmar.

Given the tremendous diversity and complexity amongst the people and administration of India, planning and implementing partition needed a great deal of organisation and thought. The power of the British Raj—profoundly domineering for nearly a century—left a political, cultural, and psychological legacy. This also meant it took tremendous pressure directed over a long period of time to build consensus that Britain needed to leave. However, the execution of this departure lacked the consideration that was required. During the review of partition in 2017, the authors learnt more about the impact that the sense of panic had on the people. This urgency was due in part to the escalating violence expressing (in our view) some of the frustrations and pressures that had accumulated amongst the people. The discounting of this crucial information may have added to the division and rage that was being acted out. As families and people became further divided, the impetus to fury escalated, resulting in what many have described as retributive genocide.

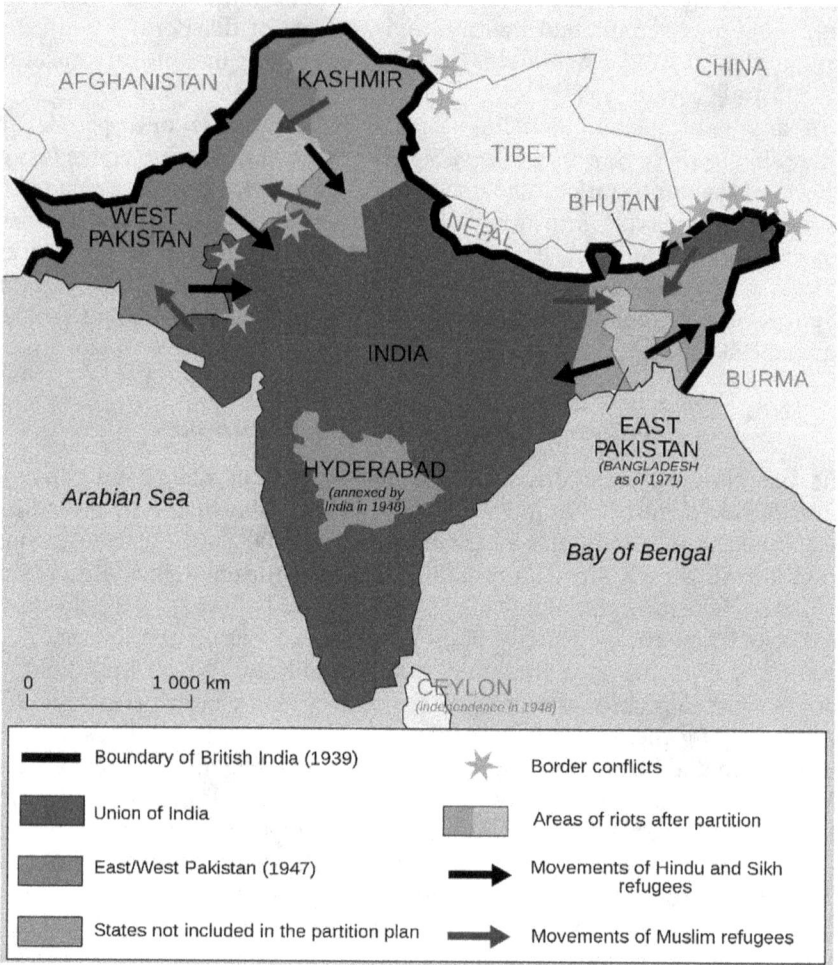

Figure 6.1 The partition of India (1947). (Image by Partage_de_l'Inde.svg, 2010, reproduced from Wikimedia Commons under CC BY-SA 3.0.).

The minimising of the significance of this escalating violent migration and the subsequent ruthless implementation of boundaries marked a generation. The Boundary Commission, led by the British lawyer Cyril Radcliffe, delivered terrible mistakes. Radcliffe later admitted that he had had to rely on out-of-date maps and census materials (BBC News, 2017). This is a short historical background, serving as a backdrop to the personal stories of both our fathers and how they have embodied their era. Our fathers were 15 and 16 when partition took place.

Farah: I remember my father telling me about listening to Ghandi and Nehru on the radio discussing the complicated politics of India and the uncertainty of the future. These times were difficult, but he remembers them with nostalgic happiness until his mother—whom he had a close bond with—died due to illness exacerbated by extreme poverty. He was 15 and the eldest of three. Her death devastated him and at the same time triggered deep rage as he tried to make sense of who was to blame for his loss. He took responsibility for his younger siblings and in this process lost his identity as a child.

Karen: My paternal grandmother died in childbirth when my father was just four. When I asked my father about it, he was rather dismissive, saying this happened to many Indian women. I was shocked by his acceptance of death and wondered, with my European mind, if it had left him longing for something maternal and constant. When I asked him about partition, he told me he had caught one of the last trains out of Delhi when he was 13 or 14, "before the butchering started". He looked directly at me as he declared, "They were my friends! I went to school with Sikh and Hindu boys—we visited each other's homes". Returning to Rawalpindi, he did not go on to tell me about the trauma of the riots that took place a couple of years later. But I imagine those riots—some of the worst that took place in the Punjab—the violence in 1947 was some of the most terrible. One horrific account I heard last year was how Sikh fathers killed their daughters to protect their honour and shield them from the capture, rape, and slavery that many women from all sides endured. To hear such stories even though historical and experienced in my imagination alone can feel overwhelming and the images intrude violently as I think of it …

It seems difficult to imagine how a nation recovers from such atrocities, let alone tries to build a new state. The birth of Pakistan was violent, and the rage and hatred left would take generations to recover from. Remembering and writing of his nation in the 1950s, my (Karen) father described the anger and rage of a country moving into its infancy:

The students blame the teachers, the teachers blame the students and the government and, above all, the government runs down the people. The tendency towards alienation is marked and I was brought to wonder if independence has meant any more to the Pakistani people than the substitution of the brown raj for the British raj.

(Hussain, 1966, p. 167)

73

Rage accompanying helplessness is the aftermath of trauma and this affected the new states across the Indian subcontinent as well as these two men. Both embodied the assault on their identity and dignity. Their internal dynamics were a confused mire added to by the complexity of dependency on their previous imperial ruler in Europe. Despite the cultural and psychological wreckage from colonialism and partition, both men did salvage something. They did survive, find work, and have families.

So, we turn now to their experiences in Britain; like many from this era, they sought refuge in the "motherland". Yet, this refuge had a complex nature and the shadow from colonial history spilt into this postcolonial period, creating a sense of alienation amongst the many that came to the UK at this time.

The Crisis of Belonging

In the context of colonialism, partition, and early postcolonial eras, there is support for the rhetoric of strength in nationalism whilst diminishing and dismissing economic, social, and political fallibility or vulnerability. Our interpretation is that this promotes "one mind thinking" (Wieland, 2015) and is defensive of any critique of the establishment as well as a denigration of philosophical, social, political, and psychological differences.

In an atmosphere where "otherness" in society and within the mind is killed off or banished, it is as if the masculine and what that might represent has to be aggrandised to protect against the risk that anything representing the feminine can make itself known. This is grounded in a White racist form of masculinity. For instance, Frantz Fanon wrote, "black is not a man" (1952/2021, p. 138) and Wieland (2015) described the Jews being portrayed as feminised men in 19th-century Germany and across Europe. It was within this mindset that our fathers lived when they came to the UK. In other words, we suggest that the earlier period of colonialism involved the subjugation and therefore emasculation of Indian men. We think this legacy contributed to a vulnerability to feeling humiliated alongside repression and dissociation of rage. We also wonder how this contributed to the dynamics in their relationships with our White mothers. There was little time for new nations to recover and rebuild after colonialism and the traumas of partition. So, at a personal level, there was little time for our fathers to adjust to the impact of being raised during the era of colonialism as well as recovering from their adolescent years where they witnessed social, political, and environmental traumas. The residue of such experiences must have been available to be ignited on arrival in Britain.

Colonialism had offered hope via education—a chance to carve a better life for oneself. Education, academic and professional qualifications continue to be seen as passports to privilege in many postcolonial countries. In the formative period from the 1950s to the 1970s, children of this era were creating social mobility, moving from the working class to the middle class. Colonial rule had meant that many men in India and Pakistan were fluent in English. The presence of the British had made many believe they understood the English people. During the 1950s and 1960s, the British government actively encouraged travel to England and, with the process being relatively straightforward, many decided to venture there and send money back home to families. Farah's father, like many, believed it was his duty to do that and he believed this would give his family hope and opportunity.

Farah: My father tried hard to transition into UK society. Even though he was a Muslim, he went to the pub, drank alcohol with English men, and exchanged "banter" with his work colleagues. He tried to integrate himself into the social norms … but it seemed as if they rejected him randomly, resulting in internal confusion and paranoid thinking. He felt this was all about his difference, his colour and ethnicity, particularly when he displayed his cultural norms or thinking. He told the story of how his Irish friend (a woman, also subjected to maltreatment and abuse for being Irish) requested out of self-protection that they walk separately on the streets. He was deeply hurt and angered by this. There were echoes here of his life in India as he was not allowed to associate with his Hindu or Sikh friends due to reprisals that could include death.

Karen: My father told one story of how he and my mother were being verbally abused for being together, when travelling on a train. With White men he often felt a heightened sense of alienation. He found reception with women, and he forged many friendships—some sexual, some intellectual, and some both. Some aspects of his curiosity about people and the meaning of his experiences remained alive; he had a capacity to think philosophically and was available in part to the language of feelings and their importance in belonging and identity. From humble beginnings he carved, at least for a short time in his adult life, something of a productive life. Like many countries that were colonised, education for some children in India and Pakistan was a path out of poverty. Whilst this describes his better self, it is not the whole picture and his capacity to collapse under pressure and become oppressive and aggressive on occasion meant there were many fragmented and destructive features to his life.

Highlighting or emphasising difference and protecting identity to some degree enabled my (Karen) father to continue thinking. He somehow managed to hold on to his mind by understanding and following an academic path. The translation of experience into knowledge might have marked a determination in his professional life to overcome haunting memories and to try to discover some hope. The connections he made at the India Club in London helped him forge friendships and alliances that encouraged his thinking capacity and a continuation of his identity whilst here in London.

Perhaps both fathers knew they had to transition well, and they each had a personal determination to escape their troubled land and survive. Their hurt came from being rejected by the same ethnic group, the English, who had divided and fragmented their country, leaving it a place of loss, death, and grief. The 2018 controversy in the UK, the "Windrush scandal", has led to many men and women originally from the Caribbean being targeted by the Home Office because they were missing a British passport. After decades of living in the UK, it has been shocking to see that, like our fathers, they had wrongly believed that they would be welcome and protected in England. These experiences evoke strong feelings of betrayal and our fathers responded to this in their individual ways.

Farah: My father felt duped by the British Government and society; this fed a kind of primitive distrust of the English. He learnt that English men would say one thing to your face but have completely different responses in private—they had two faces ... He used to use the expression "double faced" from a very hurt place. When he returned to Pakistan he was revered by his family and friends because he had "made it" and appeared, relative to their poverty, as incredibly wealthy and educated. This "new" English filter and his experiences of London meant that he had further introjected a sense of British supremacy and so looked upon some of the cultural behaviours and mentality of his relatives as backward, less than. His one-up, superior attitude towards them may have soothed him internally and might have been welcome respite after so much injury. I wonder also whether it was a defence against feelings of guilt and shame when faced with their relative poverty and destitution. Further, after being made to feel "small" by the English, this may have been his attempt at restoring his ego and dignity after suffering the humiliation of racism from his host country. Upon returning to London, my father was forced to continue revering the "superiority" of the "White colonial masters". Attempting to join and belong to British society fed his ego and was, we think, a narcissistic defence against the shame and humiliation that he endured.

Karen: My father tried in his professional life to find some alchemical gold, and his personal life in England was for a few years charismatic, exciting, as well as dishevelled and fragmented. He left significant trails of personal destruction behind him, which left him and others feeling alienated. Those close to him often ended up feeling angry, humiliated, or betrayed by some of the ways he conducted himself.

The losses have been profound and seem to indicate the enactments related to trauma in the aftermath of partition on his country.

The fragmentation that came about in India continues in Britain today and has been transmitted down the generations of the Sikh, Muslim, and Hindu communities. With the rise of terrorism and Islamophobia, Sikhs and Hindus are at pains to justify their differences from their Muslim "brothers and sisters" to the dominant White population as a way of protecting them from the affliction of abuse and hatred. So, with this diaspora, this trail to the West has had consequences. In particular, we point to the conflict between the need to be affirmed, to be validated by the White establishment and an anger with the vulnerability to denigration that has accompanied this need.

Consequences of Migration

The legacy of colonialism and subsequent migrations to the West has informed political and foreign policy. Global migration, and the more modern versions of voluntary diaspora have had complicated consequences politically, socially, and psychologically. We, the authors, are postcolonial children and as such we embody these experiences as well as our ancestral heritage of colonialism. As "mixed children" we have both the coloniser and the colonised in our DNA. We share some examples of how we have experienced this heritage.

Farah: I was raised around North West London which has been classified as the most ethnically diverse region in Europe. Being of mixed heritage I identify strongly with my London and French European roots. At school, I remember being shown maps of the world coloured in pink to identify the countries that had been colonised by the English. My father's interpretation was that the British had simply stolen and taken what they wanted, including the Crown Jewels with the Koh-i-Noor diamond. During Queen Elizabeth's Jubilee celebrations in the 1970s, I remember how his bitterness and trauma were activated by the parading of these jewels with no mention of how they were obtained.

I remain based in London which continues to be a multicultural environment and I sometimes wonder how the Empire exists in London. What is interesting for me is the fear that is so easily aroused and how this may have contributed to the Brexit vote. I feel a sense of pride in being the child of two successful immigrants. Later in life, I have sometimes felt forced by others—including clients—to claim an identity or to be defined by their projection. For example, being seen by some men as "exotic" and by others as "an unwelcome drain on British society". This evokes strong feelings including rage and shame for me. Whilst I have needed to develop a capacity to hold hostile projections, there have been other more benign projections—sometimes even creative ones, based on curiosity to discover something about my difference.

Karen: I was the darkest amongst my siblings. My conscious awareness of my colour really developed when we first returned to England from Nigeria, when I was ten. Here in England, I was at the receiving end of racial abuse from other children in my class. This was confusing and difficult for me, given that many of my friends in Nigeria had been Black or of mixed heritage. There I had identified with them, as well as trying to navigate my sense that I was also "White". I was seen as White in Africa, yet Black in the UK. This was complex and confusing, compounded by the different projections I was now facing. As a clinician, I have experienced sexualised objectification, curiosity, as well as racial hatred as you describe, Farah, for coming here and taking over jobs and professions. My physical presence as a woman of colour has aroused a number of conscious and unconscious processes and intersubjective dynamics. In addition, I have sometimes felt myself to be the face of the "acceptable other". In other words, my sense of being "the other" amongst colleagues as well as the adult learners poses a mild rather than a radical disturbance. I think the journey to personal and social pluralism in the UK continues to be long.

For both of us, having been raised under British hegemony has led to internal tension in our wish and our reluctance to belong. We find ourselves drawn into groups and communities and then wanting to pull away, retreat for protection and recuperation. Some of this is common for many people drawn to psychotherapy as a profession and the pull/push in us has been both conscious and unconscious. We discover more from sharing such experiences and offering our observations of each other in and out of groups. Our resistance to being dominated again and our profound need to be independent is linked to our strong urge to survive. We fear subjugation; when we reflect back on our relational experiences of it, it can feel like a death. So, the numbing, anaesthetising that Bollas (1987) wrote about in connection to extractive introjection speaks to us vividly.

As clinicians we have noticed that some clients discover permission to discuss their own differences as they see the differences in us. There is sometimes an assumption that we will understand their internal alienated world of what it is like to be different, to struggle to belong whether that be as a result of sexuality, ethnicity, or gender. So, curiosity and confusion about our ethnicity sometimes leads to a desire to connect to us socially, as real women. This has pressed us to think a great deal about how we want to hold ourselves as professionals. For instance, where our personal and professional boundaries sit in terms of personal revelations and how much we think is therapeutically helpful to either share or withhold. We are both inclined to work relationally with intersubjective psychodynamics—so we often hold tensions with our appearance and identity between both the real "I/Thou" relationship (Clarkson, 1993) as well as the transferential one.

We recognise our ambivalence around belonging resonates with the experiences of our fathers who, as we have shown, felt a deep sense of alienation after moving away from their fragmented homeland. Rather than belong, our fathers pursued nomadic lives and interests and were literally "lost between two shores" (Diamond, 1971). Like them, we have been challenged as to what to do about where we identify and feel we belong to. Sometimes we have ended up electing to be on the periphery of communities, perhaps so we can move in and out with ease and no ties.

Both our fathers were modern and liberal compared to many of their Muslim peers and we are thankful for that. It was important to them that we were educated and independent women. Within Indian culture it is the norm for parents to take an active part in their children's education, and further, to not allow their children to take their education for granted. Our fathers wanted us to have transferable skills to set up anywhere in the world, to be independent, and not reliant on others. We suggest that this is at times a tough formula, to be resourceful and flexible in order to survive. We think of this as part of the "immigrants' state of mind", a mindset in our view that emerges from the need to find life away from home because of trauma and poverty. Looking back at history and thinking currently about migration, we think this may exist globally as part of immigrants' psyches.

Nationalism—A 21st-Century Challenge

The question of how a newly born state might facilitate a new identity for its people would seemingly require a deep connection with the philosophy and psychology of belonging as well as the wisdom and capacity to bring about such an ambitious outcome. One day our fathers were Indian and then overnight they became Pakistani. A few years later and both were attempting to make a life in the UK. Barriers to thriving were numerous, whether it be in the search for lodgings, jobs, or progress in careers. Some of the examples we have shared indicate the state of mind that is evoked when there is a terrible fear of being robbed by the hated and alien "other". We suggest such states of mind attack internal possibilities for democracy, so that parochialism and totalitarian states of mind become the dominant feature.

The chaos of partition has been reflected in our process of writing this. As writers sharing experiences, we lost our way several times as free association and spontaneous reminiscing was shared. Ordering our memories and subjective experiences into a coherent narrative has been a challenge. We understood this as a powerful parallel process that mirrored something frantic about the speed of partition and the impossibility for millions of people to come to terms with what had been lost, won, and what needed to be rebuilt across the Indian subcontinent.

Across the globe, difference has evoked struggles, conflicts, fights, and splits. These have inspired wars and contributed to all manner of atrocities. The complexity of identity, including national, regional, cultural, racial, political, and psychological identities destabilise us, divide us, and challenge us to face our limitations. Needing to belong to a land, and fights to claim land, contribute to the writing and rewriting of history, geography, and culture. Add to this international, national, and regional politics that influence social identity, as well as conscious and unconscious psychological processes, and there are multiple layers at work when it comes to working in the consulting room. The global historical and revisiting phenomena of White masculine supremacy, as well as reactions and responses to this, remain a potent and complex contribution to how we live, communicate, and negotiate together. It seems that from time to time, even as much as nearly a century on, people are pushed to return to the problems encountered but not resolved by our fathers.

Notes

1 Some images captured by Margaret Bourke-White are available at https://tribune. com.pk/story/864867/11-devastating-pictures-from-the-1947-partition and https:// partitionofunitedindia.weebly.com/pictures.html
2 *Viceroy's House* is a 2017 British-Indian historical drama film directed by Gurinder Chadha and written by Paul Mayeda Berges, Moira Buffini, and Chadha. The film stars Hugh Bonneville, Gillian Anderson, Manish Dayal, Huma Qureshi, and Michael Gambon. It was selected to be screened out of competition at the 67th Berlin International Film Festival.
    The film was released in the United Kingdom on March 3, 2017, while the Hindi dubbed version titled *Partition: 1947* was released in India on August 18, 2017, three days after its 70th Independence Day. It was released worldwide on September 1, 2017. Viceroy's House is based on *Freedom at Midnight* by Larry Collins and Dominique Lapierre, and *The Shadow of the Great Game: The Untold Story of Partition* by Narendra Singh Sarila. (Wikipedia, 2022, paras. 1–2)

Part II

RADICAL-RELATIONAL REFORMATION

Introducing Part Two

Radical-Relational Reformation

The second half of this book reviews "liberation" as it was described in the 1960s and 1970s by the radical psychiatry group though from a contemporary perspective. In the original formula, liberation from oppression was the goal, the path to recovery. The idea was taken from the fights against legitimised discrimination, especially racism and sexism from that time. As such, the original idea that personal, psychological, and political liberation was linked and that contact, engagement, and purpose were the antidote to alienation was a pioneering perspective in the psychological fields. This was completely different to what had gone before, in that psychological distress had been understood as originating and residing in the individual's mind. As such, depression could be understood as a "chemical imbalance", something there-fore that could be treated medically and behavioural symptoms that could be corrected with treatments such as CBT (Cognitive Behavioural Therapy). My view is that we can turn this around and come to understand distress in all its forms very differently. Rather than the sickness seen as residing almost entirely in the individual, I am coming to understand that the individual carries the symptoms of a sick society. I have argued for a relational perspective of course in that none of us are empty vessels, so the resources we have been born with and the way these have been affected by our families and social experiences have mattered. In this respect, my interpretation is in alignment with the original manifesto: "People's troubles have their source not within them but in their alienated relationships, in their exploitation, in polluted environments, in war, and in the profit motive" (Steiner et al., 1975, p. 4).

The path to liberation was believed to create social and psychological freedom and this was challenging and direct about the work that was to be

DOI: 10.4324/9780429289231-8

done. During the writing of this book, I am frequently reminded of the protest marches in the 1960s and 1970s and the ways in which protests have continued and evolved over the decades. My experience has been that these earlier protests against social structures of racism such as apartheid in South Africa, the ongoing women's rights movement, the anti-war protests—especially one of the largest against the Vietnam war—and the many inspirational speeches, interviews, and broadcasts of that earlier era epitomised a rising in consciousness that has been returned to and built upon subsequently. This era also marked the growth in public broadcasting, and in some parts of the globe, the wider use of television meant that the pictures and stories could reach right into our families' living spaces. This has continued in exponential ways with the expanse, even explosion, of social media. This then is our/my legacy, serving as the backdrop, the context from which we/I have developed personally and professionally.

Thus, this part of the book asks: if we accept alienation as the key challenge, what is it that we need to attend to in order to heal? Is "liberation" still a valid quest? If so, what are the components that might lead to a sense of freedom, or meaning, or recovery? In the next chapter, I cite the original formula Steiner and colleagues proposed. They talked of the need for awareness that leads to anger and then the need for contact. This support can lead to action, which is the path to liberation. The language used is of its time—strident, political—a passionate call to action. In light of this, I review past and current fights against regimes as protests about political and cultural alienation.

7

FROM SOCIAL LIBERATION TO RADICAL-RELATIONAL REFORMATION

> Thus, social psychology shows us that, in order to change his character, the individual must be given a sense of purpose and a feeling of participation in the adventure of national progress. If this is not achieved, volumes of speeches will not succeed in building bridges which will enable the individual to cross from the claustrophobic atmosphere of parochialism to the wider spaces of national interest.
>
> (Hussain, 1966, p. 43)

Introduction

I start this chapter with a quote from my father's book. Written during the era of the radical psychiatry movement and the fights for social justice that I have referred to, it is a reminder of how the social, political, and psychological are relationally bound. This second half of this book considers the development from "liberation" as it was described in the 1960s and 1970s to contemporary perspectives on emancipation from oppression. In the original formula, social liberation was the goal, and the social and political pursuit of activism that led to psychological freedom. As such, the original idea that personal, psychological, and political liberation were linked and that contact, engagement, and purpose were the antidote to alienation was a pioneering perspective in the psychotherapeutic fields. This was different from the 20th-century perspective in the West that psychological distress originated and resided in the individual's mind. Whether people today have the knowledge and practice of psychoanalysis, a medical perspective about chemical imbalances, or the functional pragmatism of CBT[1], individuals still tend to be treated as individuals with personal psychopathology without enough of a wider perspective on relational perspectives of the impact of society on internal human functioning and vice versa.

As described in Chapter Two, the radical psychiatry group opposed the position that sickness resided almost entirely in the individual; they suggested the opposite—that the individual carries the symptoms of a

DOI: 10.4324/9780429289231-9

pathological society[2]. The path to liberation as described by Steiner was a cry for social liberation that comes about through activism. Steiner's writing claimed psychological freedom was gained en route through activism and this was a challenging and direct perspective about the work that was to be done. During my experience of writing this book, I have often been reminded of the ways in which protests have continued and evolved over the decades. My experience has been that earlier protests against social structures, such as apartheid in South Africa as well as in many states of the USA, the ongoing women's and gay rights movement, and the anti-war protests, epitomised a rising consciousness that continued through the decades of my life. Whilst oppressive systems continue to thrive, there have also been some inspirational speeches over the years, as well as interviews and broadcasts back then and now that provide opportunities for breakthroughs. These breakthroughs occur because people can to some extent still feel, still care, and still think. The growth in public broadcasting and the wider use of television from the second half of the 20th century meant that pictures and stories sometimes from around the world have reached right into our families' living spaces. This of course has continued in exponential ways later in the 20th century and onwards into the 21st with the expanse, even explosion of social media, which has raised the potential for individuals to broadcast incidents and news. Now, messages picked up by political pressure groups and activists such as Black Lives Matter, the inspirational Greta Thunberg, and Extinction Rebellion means information can be sent and received across the globe. This development of protesting and pressurising has been part of my legacy, serving as a backdrop, a context from which I have developed personally and professionally.

Radical Psychiatry and the Path to Liberation

In the original formula, Steiner et al. (1975) highlight the need for awareness to replace deception. In some ways, Wyckoff and her colleagues are challenging a White capitalist mindset by drawing on the feminist and anti-racist movements of the time which were raising the bar in terms of intelligent and focused protest, argument, and debate. Using the language of that era, these writers also recognise how social and psychological deception maintains the systems that hold capitalist norms in place. They describe that people need to become aware of their oppression. When people come to realise they have had "the metaphorical wool pulled over their eyes" (Minikin, 2018, p. 118) they will feel angry. The group identify that the difference between alienation and anger was awareness of the deception. They made a convincing case that psychiatry contributed to perpetuating deception by taking the view that pathology resided within the individual. Therefore, awakening the mind to deception evoked anger and was growth. It was a healthy and motivational

84

step towards liberation. Thus, in their formula, their group wrote (Wyckoff et al., 1975, p. 12):

Oppression + Awareness = Anger

Having argued that people will feel anger about deception, the radical psychiatrist group go on to argue that the motivation and energy evoked by this anger can be met and channelled productively through contact with others who have also suffered. This coming together, and contact with others who understand such anger, who care enough about it, and who want to connect, makes activism possible. Groups can organise and fight for social justice. And according to the radical psychiatry movement, it is this social and political action that creates the momentum for personal change and liberation (Steiner et al., 1975, p. 14):

Awareness + Contact = Action Liberation

The recovery from political and social alienation through action leads to liberation and represents an important and ambitious project. Widespread and powerful protests, such as the civil rights movement, the campaign for nuclear disarmament, and the associated Greenham Common Peace camp, have all required an optimistic state of mind, a feeling that outrage must land, will be heard and must have influence on that centre, the norm, and the power base. In many places, much progress was fought for and achieved through such political, social, and interpersonal contact. Ongoing mean-ingful campaigns continue, and as a political person, this feels important and I am grateful for these fights, as well as the earlier ones mentioned. In the West, such fights may symbolise what we think of as democracy—the right to protest and speak out. Yet, it is important to acknowledge that many fights, protests, and quests for liberation come at a cost. Many people have been imprisoned, tortured, and killed because they fought for what they believed in; many fought to make a better situation for the wider good and the generations to come.

This capacity of us as people to put ourselves at risk for the greater good can feel inspirational to the collective. Perhaps this goes some way to un-derstanding that the tone in the language used by the radical psychiatry manifesto is of its time. It is strident, powerful—a passionate call to action. The activist in me appreciates such feelings and such words. However, the psychotherapist that I am seeks the bridge into the consulting room. How do I find ways to help my clients with their internal worlds and the way the internal is relationally bound to the external? As such, I thought a lot about the original path to liberation and found it did not quite capture how I experienced and thought about deep structural psychological change. Was it therapeutically enough? How do social and political dynamics work as intrapsychic and intersubjective processes? If protests are one way to achieve progress out there in the world, is the same true of "in here"? In our consulting rooms, within our own minds? What is it that we need to face in terms of our internal oppressive dynamics?

Within Transactional Analysis there are some approaches, especially those that were in favour through the 1970s and 1980s, that epitomise this quest for liberation. The classical school within Transactional Analysis leans towards an analysis of ego states, transactions, games, and script. The quest is for the grown adult to find more functional ways of relating. Berne himself seemed to have shifted his position over a decade or so from an exploration of something more internal, more insight-based (Berne, 1961), to an approach that leaned towards the behavioural (Berne, 1975):

> Transactional analysis is a theory of personality and social action, and a clinical method of psychotherapy, based on the analysis of all possible transactions between two or more people on the basis of specifically defined ego states, in a finite number of established types (nine complementary, 72 crossed, 6480 duplex and 36 angular).
>
> (p. 20)

Perhaps the need for behavioural change was indicative of the optimism of the time: classical Transactional Analysis advocated efficiency—a type of *change now, analyse later* philosophy. This was built upon by the redecisional school who, drawing on the work of Fritz Perls, advocated the therapist to step away from, or even confront directly, transferential experiences. Their methodology included returning to the literal and actual memory of the original pain and reliving it often through a kind of psychodrama so that new outcomes and perspectives can be achieved. This tended to empower the Child over the oppressive Parent. The difficulty for me in these approaches is an overemphasis on "reality", or what the conscious mind can draw up, recall, and report to the therapist. My experience has been that this lends itself to cognitive processing, which seems not enough. Furthermore, my experience as a client has been that on occasion I needed to adapt to the therapist, who seemed convinced of the value in two-chair work and who seemed to hold a perspective of the "correct" outcome. The focus on change represents a quest for freedom from the oppression of script—a seductive notion perhaps. The draw for me with the ideas of alienation and possible recovery from this perhaps speaks more to my earlier life as a political teenager when I had felt some excitement about change, speaking out in protest, and a connection with groups of like-minded people. I could relate to what the theory described and so as a trainee in psychotherapy, alienation pointed to a particular type of consciousness raising. One that could represent something more vital, more sustainable for me. Paying attention to deception created by power dynamics offered me scope to stay awake to something.

However, the path to liberation, as described by Steiner, focuses on the social and political rather than the psychological. As a result, there was much that got discounted. For example, I am not sure there was enough acknowledgement of the risks and the costs of engaging in social and political activism. Many activists have lost livelihoods, families, or their actual physical life by taking such stands. Finding ways to uncover hidden oppression at systemic levels is a real challenge when we are all affected by normative mindsets and an innate human desire to survive and belong. Whilst activism may offer the individual a "sense of purpose" (Hussain, 1966, p. 43), I am not convinced it helps the individual to build internal bridges from totalitarian states of mind to something more flexible and democratic. To explore these ideas further, I draw on the sociological and the psychoanalytical.

The Sociological and the Psychoanalytical

From the second half of the 20th century, a wide and deep canon of academic and artistic work (see, for example, Fanon, 1952/2021) has helped to deconstruct the legacy and impact in the West of living within a White, masculine heteronormative mindset. There is growing recognition of how this is dominant, systemically speaking, with evidence that manifests through institutions, society, culture, and politics. As I am writing here in the UK, there has been scandalous revelation of racism at Yorkshire County Cricket Club (BBC Sport, 2021). Many of us who know and love the game of cricket have been aware of the embedded racism in the game and some players have spoken out about their experiences (see, for example, Holding, 2021 and Riley, 2010). Whilst the West Indian cricket team of the late 1970s and early 1980s were famous for fighting back and speaking out, the Black and Asian players that were beginning to represent England did not have the solidarity of a group. Isolated and individual members of a predominately White team have had to dig deep over the years to find resilience and strength to sustain them in what has continued to happen behind closed doors.

Today, the changes in the law and the rise of political correctness have made explicit expressions of racism, sexism, homophobia, and other forms of abuse unfashionable. In terms of the grip and hold that prejudice can have, there has been some loosening around the edges and some progress through the decades. And yet, a predominately White, heterosexual, masculine, privileged power base continues to draw favour collectively. For instance, the right-wing government in the UK and those of a similar disposition voted into power in other countries is validation that conservative populism still has a powerful hold, especially during times of economic and/

or social difficulties. Some progress has been meaningful and has been integrated into local cultures. This is more than a nod to marginalised communities. Yet, in the UK cabinet of 2021, 65% went to private school (Cowburn, 2020), though only 6.5% of children in the UK go to private school. I mention this because it indicates that the life experience of most people in the UK is not subjectively known by the people voted to represent them. So, despite democratic elections, the political and economic decision making is determined by a powerful minority, and this has influence on the social, cultural, and therefore ethical mindset of the people. In normal circumstances, this current UK government would privilege the economy, like many other nations, but the COVID-19 pandemic has forced the issue of social care and international co-operation, and possibly created some space for wider political and philosophical questions that are urgent to address, such as climate change. The irony of this being that the need to focus on health and social care follows a decade of policies focusing on austerity. Hence, in response to the pandemic, there has had to be something of a "u-turn".

In her recent book on social policy, Williams (F. Williams, 2021) refers to Raymond Williams (R. Williams, 1977) and his idea of "structures of feelings". This describes how people in the community start to think and live differently in response to the material and relational circumstances around them. Fundamentally, this affects their values, their mindsets, and sentiments that are often counter to the dominant ways. In other words, it is possible to see how sectors of the community have changed ahead of government policy. There are many examples of this in the UK, from intercultural and racial marriages to same-sex marriages and families, to queer, trans, and variant gender relations. This illustrates a different way of thinking about democracy. In other words, life, feelings, and values can change at grass roots levels and the politicians have to play catch up. Williams (F. Williams, 2021) goes on to describe an ethics which is grounded in a mindset of care, the environment, and decoloniality. She states that "morality and politics are not separate spheres but entwined through an understanding of the social relations of power" (F. Williams, 2021, pp. 174–175). Given the parallels for what I am arguing for as an approach in psychotherapy, I will refer back to this in my final chapter.

Learning from the fields of sociology helps to gain some academic backup to what I have been thinking about and working with from my education in counselling and psychotherapy and my life experience. That is the relationality between the social, political, and economic structures that provide a context from which we have been raised and how this relates and interacts with our personal and internal resources and worlds. Our social structures have allowed us to grow, to develop, to know who we are, and to get engaged, validated our contributions, as well as inhibited or even traumatised us in these areas. These experiences are our legacies and contribute to our identities. It has meant some of us have had to struggle or fight some more to contribute and engage with our communities and social responsibilities. These experiences contribute to resilience as well as our vulnerabilities and our frailties.

In linking the philosophical with sociology and psychoanalysis, I have found much to value in the writing of Fromm (1956, 1962). Fromm, like the radical psychiatry group of his era, considers both Marx and Freud. He takes Marx's thinking about alienation, and applying this to his insight as a psychoanalyst he considers the fractures within the human mind. In this sense he makes a case for alienation as the root cause in manifesting neurosis:

> In the widest sense, every neurosis can be considered an outcome of alienation; this is so because neurosis is characterized by the fact that one passion (for instance, for money, power, women, etc.) becomes dominant and separated from the total personality, thus becoming the ruler of the person.
>
> (Fromm, 1962, p. 43)

Fromm was progressive in challenging the masculine power base as early as the 1950s and 1960s. He picks up that masculinity is being defined in terms of capitalist values. He is pointing to the sort of defence that encourages a disavowal of vulnerability. Although writing decades earlier than Wieland (2015), I see the connection between what he said then and what she writes about in the 21st century:

> To be a boy ... was to be constantly threatened with castration— unmanning, emasculation, feminisation ... I suggest that the castration complex is Freud's major contribution to the understanding of masculinity—its precariousness, its ambivalence about mother/woman ...
>
> (Wieland, 2015, p. 63)

These quotes remind me of Alan's story that I introduced the reader to in Chapter Three. So, drawing on contemporary writers, as well as my personal and professional experiences, I continue to search for a contemporary and relational way to address the experience of alienation. I retain the perspective that deception is key in its capacity to retain power imbalances, dependency, and passivity, all of which collude with normative structures. So, it seems important to understand this further. Normativity allows people to internalise deception and buy into the values and norms of the power base. This means our minds continue to facilitate oppression by defending against seeing how we are being oppressed. To comprehend how we are being oppressed must therefore be disturbing. Separating our minds from those we love and from the power base of the communities and societies we live in risks our sense of

89

belonging. The implications are that we need regular reminders to stay awake and to keep our minds active and alive, so that we do not become deadened and collusive to the seduction (Minikin, 2021) of normativity.

A Personal Illustration: "Almost White"

A year ago, I was due to present on a panel that was, in part, to debate the dynamics of difference in the consulting room. The keynote speaker was a man of dual heritage whose skin tone and colour were similar to mine. A week before the event, I had a dream.

In my dream, I created the scenario of the panel. The keynote speaker was alongside three women: me and two others, both of whom were White (although they also had life experiences and feelings about being marginalised, albeit different from my own). The audience members, which included some familiar faces and some strangers, were full of passion and shouting with all their might: "They look Italian! They are almost White!" It was a vital, vivid dream, and on waking I was somewhat startled by the image. I asked myself: "Why was I having such a loud dream? Why does it matter? What might my dream have been pointing to?"

Perhaps I was negotiating something about my relationship to race and authority, and my feelings and position with those. Most of my colleagues and community acquaintances are White, as are many of my friends. I also have colleagues, clients, supervisees, friends, and family who are Black, Asian, and mixed race, but White people are in the majority in my current day-to-day life. So, to find myself in a position of authority with another who also mirrored something of my heritage was stirring my conscious and unconscious mind and registering as something significant and impactful. I was being pushed to face up to something because of the novelty of that mirroring for me. I was preparing myself for my visibility and the unusual position of holding authority with a largely White audience. I was actively wondering how we would be received.

I was struck that my dream image spoke to my potential anxiety about that exposure. My hope was that we would be listened to, related to, and allowed to speak because, after all, we were really just a little bit brown. I think it is true that a little bit brown evokes less racism than very Black. So, was my dream picking up on that dynamic? It was also one of the points the keynote speaker spoke about in relation to his clinical work (Hart, 2022). That is, between people of colour, especially those who have an experience of inter- and/or transgenerational trauma associated with race—and, particularly in this example, shadeism—there is an awareness and sensitivity to how dark or fair your colour is. Perhaps I was trying to grasp some comfort, a kind of reassurance that I was not going to be alone with this; someone else knew, experienced, and lived with this particular dynamic. As with all dreams, there is always much more that could be said, looked at, and taken from it, but for the purposes of this chapter, it made me think further about the desire to belong, accompanied by the inclination to minimise difference.

Desire to Belong

Interpersonal and intersubjective theories such as Transactional Analysis make it clear how vulnerable we are to influence from the outside. The outside will respond to our outsides. Our exterior, visible selves have to "take" what comes our way and process it, deal with it, or absorb and/or defend against it. Our reactions and responses will depend on our state of mind, our sense of self, our moment-by-moment groundedness—or lack thereof. When we are conscious of a visible identity that is different from or diminished by the societal norm, we may well have personal conscious or unconscious dilemmas: Do we go with a felt longing to belong, or do we hold our difference with confidence, pride, or even rebellion? Inevitably, belonging defines a group, and in doing so it also defines the exclusions from that group. I suggest that when there have been profound experiences of trauma and oppression, self-protective defences promote a diminishing of parts of the self, a withholding, a retreat in some cases, a splitting off from relatedness with that difference in an effort to survive or thrive in the presence of the more powerful other.

So, in a society in which the norm for power holding is White, male, and middle-aged, alternative authority figures may stir up interesting processes for all parties. If we accept that our desire to be seen as normal is a fundamental one and that we need to belong, it follows that all parts of our identity are relative in relation to what is perceived as the majority. In the West, we have seen some efforts in recent decades to have different identities represented publicly, such as having diverse individuals represented as role models (e.g., Black and disabled news readers, famous faces coming out, intersex and trans-educative TV programs, etc.). Simultaneously, there has been a backlash: the young are seeking extreme ways to modify difference in pursuit of what is seen as perfection (Orbach, 2019). So, we may lean into our advantaged identities to exist—be received, heard, and respected—and to avoid the pain of exclusion and discrimination, which is essentially a rejection, an expression of hate. I call this minimising of marginality and amplifying of normativity "relative privilege".

Relative Privilege: Benefits and Costs

Returning to my dream, the feelings were passionate and hopeful in some ways. They suggested a way of relating between the speakers and the audience, of finding things in common, a degree of physical mirroring, values, and a mindset that could be reached and understood. We, the panel, with the audience might have an opportunity to "be" together, to recognise that familiarity helps us to empathise.

91

Simultaneously, my dream represented a compromise, an illustration of how marginalised selves negotiate their presentation to the norm or mainstream. And I do not restrict my point to race. To a larger or lesser extent, all marginalised identities have a relationship of dependency to the mainstream. With that, people such as me who are of mixed heritage may wonder from time to time about "getting away with it", that is, passing as White. For others it may include passing as straight, cis, able-bodied, able-minded, or all sorts of other norms against which we measure ourselves and may, at times, experience ourselves to be wanting.

Another way of thinking about this is a compromise position of "almost OK". I want to emphasise that this position is not invented by the marginalised identity. Rather, it is put upon them by the mainstream. On the larger political dimension, some identities are acceptable, others less so. Acceptability of identities is amplified by the visibility and voice of authority figures: those who have the capacity to influence societal structures and processes as well as people's mindsets. Dalal (2012) questionned the liberal narratives of inclusivity and tolerance and invited us to examine the limits of who and what is tolerable or intolerable to us. In so doing, he has examined the ways in which tolerance operates at macro and individual levels. Among the dynamics I have observed in mainstream culture are the ways in which identities can be just about tolerated as long as they do not become the norm. As long as such groups stay on the margins and know their place, for example: "I am fine that you are gay as long as you don't kiss in front of me, rub my nose in it. Keep yourself understated. Then I don't have to be disturbed by my own feelings. I don't have to evoke my ostracising tendencies. In fact, I might talk to you, even manage to be your friend and hang out with you. In return, you need to see me as a tolerant, accepting, and generous other".

This, I suggest, points to the way in which psychological collusion may operate. The powerful other offers the benefits of almost "OKness", and the marginalised subject accepts that position along with the costs. In other words, the power base offers inclusion and belonging as long as this does not deconstruct and threaten the norm. It is the powerbase, the norm, that gets to bestow or withhold "OKness". The less powerful subject can experience internal vulnerability that is associated with the marginalised identity. So, it may feel tempting to be seduced and pulled into accepting this dynamic. I suggest this process creates confusion or mystification for individuals (Steiner et al., 1975) about their own identity or multiple identities. Without protection of their more vulnerable part self, the subject is open to seduction into believing that as long as they minimise their "otherness", the longed-for acceptance and relatedness really is on offer.

The cost accompanying the acceptance of almost "OKness" is anxiety conscious and/or unconscious because the powerful other retains control of bestowing or withdrawing their gift. I am reminding the reader of the symbiotic bind that I wrote about in Chapter Four. The full sense and vitality of some identities, especially the more oppressed ones, cannot be fully experienced. With conditional acceptance, there is always the accompanying risk of rejection. It can be called upon in a moment. The subject is therefore vulnerable to losing their own volition and self-acceptance. I argue this is, in part, because the other (mainstream/ norm) has done that to them, and it works because the subject holds a natural desire to belong and be accepted. Thus, they let differentiation go and buy into mainstream values. Perhaps this offers a beginning. A way of trying to understand why it takes decades and decades for the social and psychological to marry up. As Layton (2020) challenges:

> The historical moment offers a good chance for us and our profession to wake up. We've had such opportunities before, and we didn't go there. Indeed, if anyone in dominant psychoanalytical institutions had listened to Fromm and Fanon ... in the 1950s and 1960s, I'd probably not have to argue, these many years later, that psychotic process is permeated by history and social circumstance.
>
> (p. 273)

With a relational and integrative psychotherapy, psychoanalysis offers scope to explore deeply within, whilst sociology and its social analysis offers the capacity to look out, systemically. As a relational Transactional Analyst, I draw from both in order to consider how we might find a path that includes the radical and the relational.

The Relational and Radical

The relational bond with families, communities, and our environment creates tension systemically as well as within individuals. The relational paradigm shifted the psychoanalytical one-person perspective (Stark, 1999) to an inter-subjective dynamic. The psychoanalytical and the intersubjective elements were missing in some of the earlier radical writing. As Cornell (2020) writes:

> For Steiner it seems that the causes of games and script, the forces of injunctions, attributions, alienation and oppression, remained those of the outside acting upon and against the individual. The forces of one's own unconscious, of one's own distorted thinking and projections, and of personal vulnerabilities rarely seemed to occupy a place within Steiner's thinking.
>
> (p. 79)

This is a valid and important critique and draws attention to the resources we have been born with, our subsequent experiences, and the way these have been dealt with internally. There is a complex ebb and flow between defences, homeostasis, and psychological and social change. Systemic and radical change at social and political levels is not easy; it is often traumatic. The same could be said of internal psychic change, it can hurt—a lot. So, in bringing the relational into the radical I seek to account for the relevance of the internal world, as Cornell points out, as well as account for the "sick society" (Fromm, 1962), in terms of what the individual reveals of the system and the impact on their internal world and capacity for relatedness. In this respect, I aim to explore the point made by Cornell and the analysis in Fromm's writing:

> Freud is primarily concerned with individual pathology, and Marx is concerned with the pathology common to a society and resulting from the particular system of that society ... Freud sees pathology essentially in the failure to find a proper balance between the Id and Ego ... Marx sees the essential illness as ... the estrangement of man from his own humanity and hence from his fellow man.
>
> (Fromm, 1962, p. 45)

Fromm's writing reflects a socially informed psychoanalytical perspective. He poses the questions about how to think about the cause and cure of human pain. He brings in the difference in language. Do we think of pain as psychological pathology or estrangement from our humanity? Although he was drawing on the historical writings of Marx, Fromm may have been ahead of his time in his wisdom and insight into the psychoanalytical field. It was a cross-discipline exercise that was radical because it looked outside of the medical model. Freud was keen for his theories to be accepted by medicine and in that respect psychoanalysis and subsequently psychotherapy have continued to struggle with being the poorer cousins of "proper" medical psychiatry. They have stayed on the margins, and this has, in my view, led to the enormous underresourcing and misalignment that seems to be a part of psychotherapy's script. It is so much a feature of psychotherapy services in the UK, as I wrote about in Chapter Three.

Taking the deadly dynamics of mystification, I wanted to understand better how such "mystification" or "deception" is replaced with "awareness" in the radical relational formula. How do we gain motivation to move out of an oppressive social or psychic system? Given what I have said earlier about the role of dependency and pacification in oppressive social and psychic systems, how is energy galvanised and how is independence generated? I have described the need to survive in context, so there may be much investment in submission. Therefore, it must take considerable provocation to disturb an oppressed and passive mindset.

I have written (Minikin, 2018, pp. 118–119) that some life events or contact within a therapeutic experience may provoke necessary disturbance in a stable yet oppressed psychic system. For instance, the death of a close relative, the birth of a baby, a partner's affair, the transitions of developmental growth, as well as political and social change such as the civil war experienced by many immigrants and refugees, are real life events that potentially destabilise an individual's psyche. This may leave people feeling that they do not have adequate resources to manage these disturbances alone. Minikin and Tudor (2015) wrote about the importance of developing emotional literacy (Steiner, 1997) through a co-creative and relational commitment on the part of the therapist to be profoundly engaged, affected, and willing to shift their perspectives. This is crucial to the work and can encourage an awakening of dormant subjective experiences in both parties. Therefore, engagement and participation are essential in challenging the deadening impact of oppression with deception. Hence, I propose:

Oppression + Deception + Engagement = Awakening + Disturbance

"Contact" in the original formula denoted social support from other like-minded people. This may be important in some situations. In psychotherapy, I think of contact as providing a potential container (Bion, 1959) so that the distressed person can begin to process what has happened to them. The therapist oscillates between holding (Winnicott, 1953) and containing alongside challenge and provocation to defensive and possibly destructive psychic systems. So, the quality of contact I think of in psychotherapy is more of a sense of psychological and embodied engagement (W. Cornell, personal communication, November 11, 2021) with the intersubjective process. This is not always easy and there have been many occasions when under psychic assault I have disengaged or dissociated. My point here is not that I as therapist am compelled and capable of engaging and processing all that comes to me; rather, I aim to be alive to my capacity for participation, as well as open and thoughtful about my capacity to disengage and dissociate.

Engagement then highlights the need for the therapist to be awakened and able to use their vulnerability and/or countertransference if in the service of the work. This relational dynamic, as I understand it, requires me to be available to change (Kriegman & Slavin, 1998). This is a particular version of relational working that I think is critical in a radical-relational approach. It draws on a two-person psychology (Stark, 1999) and radical openness (Hart, 2017). Here, I wish to emphasise the openness of the therapist to their own fallibilities, vulnerabilities, and aggression. Some of this may manifest consciously and some unconsciously through transference, dreams, and enactments. I also want to acknowledge that some of what the therapist is doing can be oppressive. A common way that this occurs is when we use our theory and skills to protect our egos by seeing pathology as residing almost entirely in our client. Given the philosophical premise of this book, this is the antithesis of what I hope to do. However, having been at the receiving end of this from colleagues, supervisors, and therapists on occasion, I also have to acknowledge that I have defended myself in this way when I have not had the resources to do much else. This is a challenging and necessary idea for me to bear in mind, given my commitment to anti-oppressive practice.

Over the years, I have gained some seniority in my professional community which has supported me in having a voice. However, it also means I have some experiences I am less accustomed to handling and I have had to learn as I go, so to speak. These new experiences are not so familiar from my earlier life. For example, in my community I am generally known, I have the privilege of walking into a room and people knowing my name. Having written a little, people may have the expectation that what I say is valid, possibly worth listening to. These experiences affect my work, especially as a supervisor and trainer, where there is more possibility that I will be known for the authority I have gained. To facilitate the learning and growth of others, I have at times needed to hold myself back. Not out of the need to protect myself from attacks as I may have feared as a younger woman, but because it has become easier for me to fill the space with my mind. These are the sorts of privileges that need some mindful reflection in all sorts of areas in an effort to collaborate and support learning and development for others.

Clinical Example: Dani

Many years ago, I worked with a transgender woman who was traumatised by violent attacks directed at them. They had a friendly relationship with some of the staff in a local wine bar and occasionally enjoyed going there in the evening. These outings usually ended with verbal abuse and/or violence from some of the local men. These accounts shocked and touched me deeply. Part of my shock was that we lived in a quiet town, and I had not personally encountered the sorts of assaults or attacks that were more commonplace in the streets of my younger years. I wanted to offer protection and was unsure how to talk about this without suggesting that Dani become a recluse.

The urge to protect is in part a natural human and compassionate response to another person's vulnerability. Yet, socially and psychologically I had disconnected and was experiencing myself as without resources to help. Socially, Dani was describing the kinds of assaults I had witnessed and feared as a younger woman. This connection seemed out of reach and without relevance in the moment. It was as if being so grounded now in my "cis" identity I had never known vulnerability, fear, and the threat of violence from men on the streets. It seemed as if my political and psychological insight about masculinity, its frailties, and reactions to threat were of no use when faced with the horror of Dani's story. A sense of impotent anger and helplessness engulfed us both. My expressions of shock, regret, and concern seemed empty words and I felt the urge to seek something more vital, to find something I could say or do that would make a concrete difference.

I took the situation to supervision, hoping that we might discover some answers. My supervisor took an active interest in the case. They caught my anger and desperation to help—a desperation at the time that was stuck in the social, the pragmatic, and my anger at the social injustice of it all. My supervisor started to enquire about Dani's appearance and whether they were convincing as a woman. At this point I dropped into a highly confused state. And then I became shocked when my supervisor suggested I might help my client with advice on make-up. This stalled our progress in supervision, and I left feeling disoriented, bewildered, and knowing that advice on make-up was definitely not going to be an option for me.

I think of this clinical situation as an enactment (Stern, 2010) and a parallel process (Searles, 1955). One where it was not possible for either myself or my supervisor to think socially and psychologically about what was happening. Socially, my supervisor and I were leading fairly comfortable lives at the time. So, this story of violence occurring—out there on our streets punctured our safer world, delivering the unpalatable and an impulse in both of us to find a way of making it stop. A valid enough urge, though the feelings behind it stopped us thinking like psychotherapists, stopped us holding our professional frame. We became deadened to something because we were hearing about trauma of the sort we had become ill-accustomed to dealing with in our day-to-day lives. My supervisor had resorted to suggesting I help my client to pass as "cis". We had both experienced a loss of mental structure (Bollas, 1987) as described in extractive introjection. We had both become infected by normative thinking and missed an opportunity to deconstruct our process (Derrida, 1967). Had we been able to think this through, we might have identified some important questions. For instance, what is it that needs to be attended to at a social level? What actions had been taken? What actions had not been taken? What was the impact of this on my client's confidence and identity as a transwoman? What was it like for them to leave the relative safety of a man's body and encounter the world as a transwoman? What were they hoping from me both as a "cis" woman and as a therapist? What was their relationship with protection—both as a boy, as a man, and now as transwoman? How was the vulnerability of a "cis" woman and a transwoman coming together in the consulting room? Who, if anyone, could be trusted with this experience and with protection? Exploring some of these questions may lead to some important insights, such as how easy it is to adapt to the normative frame of reference, and how normative mindsets shut off other more open and explorative ways of thinking about difficulties at a social and psychological level. We had unconsciously become oppressive by our mindset and assumed that the responsibility for protection resided with the victim of a crime rather than the perpetrator, the community, the workers in the wine bar, or even the police.

As I look back on the case and think about my supervisor's sophisticated knowledge, experience, and open-mindedness, I realise there must have been other dynamics at work. It is certainly the case that the wider social psychology includes relational and social traumas, and such dissociative processes as we were experiencing perpetuate deep adaptations to the norm. We were caught up in a collective dynamic that was bigger than our individual psychologies. Listening to the violence and abuse that my client was suffering was traumatic, and it was hard to understand and deconstruct the psychology of what was happening in the wider social realm.

Dani's exposure to hatred and the wish to kill off gender marginality left them traumatised. To have embarked on a make-up lesson would have robbed them of developing social identity and the inherent gains and losses that accompanied that. In other words, sublimation to normative structures would have potentially repressed or killed off affective experience in the way that Bollas described when the psychic life in one party is subsumed by the process in another. With my client, the parallel loss of mental structure would follow, and I believe I would have invited a diminishing sense of self. My despair as a therapist was that I would never be able to protect them from attack, and I needed to learn that was not my job. This is not to undermine the value of exploring themes of protection. However, my job was to see if it was possible for them and me to bear the level of hatred and abuse that was targeted at them. Socially, they faced men who disavowed their femininity and vulnerability, and this left their vulnerability unprotected. Our psychological job was to help keep and hold on to their own mind and grieve the loss of protection they might have had if they had stayed a man. To have worked more in this arena would have helped disturb Dani's defence against loss. Dani was tall and had a strong physique. This meant there was a dilemma to face. Whether to forego the physical safety of being visibly a man and move into the life and body that felt more true and less alienated from within but more alienating in terms of the social experience.

For clients, the experience of protection, empathy, and attunement as described in the work of Clark (1991), Erskine (1993), and Hargaden and Sills (2002) can offer an experience of feeling understood, supported, and related to. This in itself can do a lot to lower defences, though, by providing an atmosphere of trust and safety. In my experience, radical therapeutic change has also included an experience of pressure or provocation to the defensive system. Although I am drawing on the basic idea of optimal anxiety (Yerkes & Dodson, 1908), the experience of ruptures, games, and enactments do not always feel "optimal!"

Radical-Relational Reformation

Engagement may mean making demands on the subjective worlds of both client and therapist, pushing both parties to find new resources and new experiences. Through this process, oppressive frames of reference have the opportunity to get shaken. The experience of engagement allows opportunity for a breakthrough from fixated alienated states of mind to one where movement, and therefore growing resilience, becomes possible. The need for another's mind to stretch us, challenge us, and provoke us may wake us up to something. The experience of this is what I was aiming to capture when I added *awakening* + *disturbance* as part of the process; the description of what it is like to wake up to something. Even if what we are noticing for the first time is welcome, it may still be disturbing to the psyche as new information which helps create breakthroughs for client and therapist.

These awakenings and the disturbances that may accompany them represent the sense, as Kriegman and Slavin (1998) put it, that something "new" is occurring, something "genuine". Client and therapist are provoked into making use of new or unexpected self-parts and if there is enough of a genuine and stretching dynamic here on both parts, a relational connection begins, and in the fullness of time and ongoing encounters there is opportunity to experience a developing plurality with self and others. Hence, I envisaged a goal, albeit an idealistic one, of radical-relational reformation:

Awakening + Relational Connection = Plurality with Self and Others

Plurality is a state of mind that I refer to as democratic (Minikin, 2018). It is a state of mind that also links to community, to people that can tolerate strong feelings and make meaning of them without collapsing. This gives rise to a capacity to explore different states of mind in ourselves and others without defensive manoeuvres, dissociation, and/or impulsive reacting. Such engagement states help expand our relational experiences with each other and venture into new psychic territory. Socially and psychologically, this is important. It leads to being able to work together—to having allies socially and psychologically without needing to dominate, diminish, or, worse, metaphorically kill someone off or kill off some state of mind. I have come to think about the outcome of these dynamics as being twofold.

The first is reclamation of what has been lost (see Chapter Eight). In the next chapter, I go on to explain that this refers to the aspects of self and relational experiences that have been banished. Whilst a reclamation of these psychic landscapes does not mean a return to the exact same state as before, the insight of what has been lost and a grieving for that loss allows for some recovery to return to the mind and body.

The second potential outcome I describe in Chapter Eight is resurrection (see also Chapter Nine). Here, I refer to the parts of us that have been killed off or dissociated from. These refer to our responses to relational and event-based trauma. I am interested in how psychotherapy can bring renewed life and psychic energy. There is of course a genuine risk of grandiosity with such a claim. Reclamation and resurrection have enormous social, political, and religious connotations. Nonetheless, I take the risk. The original radical manifesto talked at length about "soul healing". It is the meaning of psychotherapy[3]. So, in their original statement, the spiritual met the political. In my use of the term, I refer to what the words symbolise in terms of our global and community legacy. This refers to our ancestral history, our recent histories of oppression and trauma, as well as the ongoing life experiences that affect our psychologies on a daily basis. I will continue this discussion in the following chapters.

Notes

1 See Chapter Three on the 21st-century rise of CBT.
2 The references to Fromm (1956, 1962) will come shortly. The radical psychiatry group did not reference him or others who were engaged in similar paradigms.
3 With thanks to Keith Tudor (personal communication, November 9, 2002) for pointing out the origins of this Greek word.

8

RECLAMATION
Coming Out of Exile

Introduction

Berne recognised that there was a pressing need for people to re-experience their early formative life. He gave tremendous thought to that and offered insight as to how early, and key experiences in a person's life get re-enacted in their interpersonal relations. The origin of these dynamics were the meanings the child had made of the quality of relating in their earlier life and how they had figured out the best way to survive and/or get along.

> A child's job is to find out what his parents really mean. This helps to maintain their love, or at least their protection, or in difficult cases, his mere survival. But beyond that, he loves his parents, and his chief aim in life is to please them (if they will let him), and in order to do that he has to know what they really want.
>
> (Berne, 1975, p. 101)

So, Berne referred to this as script and the re-enactments were explained as "transference drama" (Berne, 1961, p. 164). Games reflect transference dramas and were manifestations of segments of scripts played out interpersonally. Script then can be considered as a complex construction of preconscious meaning that helps the person to navigate the dynamics of relating and surviving in the context in which they live. Although script is the creative outcome of learning, perception, and evaluation, it is also defensive and there has been a price to pay for building it. Classical Transactional Analysts traditionally focused on supporting clients out of script and into more autonomous ways of being and functioning. Relational Transactional Analysts would engage with and encounter the transference drama in pursuit of understanding the emotional quality of script and allowing opportunity for transformational experiences. Both approaches value the significance of raising consciousness and grieving the loss of love. As Berne describes in the quote opening this chapter, the creation of script is an act of love, yet the compromise to my mind is the simultaneous and ironic loss of love.

DOI: 10.4324/9780429289231-10

Contributing a radical mindset to scripts means an inclusion of the relevance of social context, culture, and power dynamics. To this end, Sedgwick (2021) offers some valuable ways of thinking about script and critiquing it as a concept alongside frame of reference. He argues that script confines the individual rather too much to their own internal defensive structure, whereas frame of reference encompasses something broader and is an idea that perhaps is more open to being stretched by new ways of thinking, imagining, and dreaming, albeit this requires the mind of another, such as a therapist, arguing, "It would help us as clinicians to distinguish between occasions when insight is what is needed and those where learning about the world may be the more fruitful avenue" (Sedgwick, 2021, p. 131).

Sedgwick continues: "The appeal of the concept of frame of reference is that it brings wider questions of the usefulness, relevance, appeal and availability of belief back into the picture" (p. 133).

It does seem possible that frame of reference offers scope for thinking and encountering experience across different states of mind (or ego states as we may refer to them in Transactional Analysis). Sedgwick also describes the ongoing mutual influence at work, that contributes to the frame of reference:

> Any honest appraisal of an average person's world view will conclude that this is a kindly overestimation. Our minds also contain outdated assumptions, mistakes, errors of judgment and comprehension, tall tales and self-serving lies we have credulously taken in from similarly misguided others, vague impressions and crass generalisations, forgotten facts and inaccurate predictions. These sometimes hang together as much by the grace of god as they do by machinic efficiency.
>
> (Sedgwick, 2021, p. 134)

This is a reminder of the ongoing dynamics of alienation that capture power dynamics determining who gets to tell the truth. Sedgwick does not directly address power dynamics here, in the way that I endeavour, though he is acknowledging the challenge of finding "truth" in terms of having a position of integrity. To my way of thinking and working, I wish to stay closer to a radical and relational mindset in order to examine the relationship between alienation and recovery. So, the process of alienation diminishes love by creating the environment where inevitably unconditional love has to be foregone. Yet, the need to love lives on, but is compromised by the necessity to create a script. I interchange the process of alienation with scripting as formulating a script will include the experiences of oppression + deception. In other words, there is a need to understand and internalise the power base, buy into it out of a need to belong, and find a way of navigating the family and social system. Scripting includes the feelings of loss and a retreat or diminishing of the part of the self who loves. In other words, scripting creates the need to banish self-parts in order to protect relationships and the sense of self within the social and cultural context.

Process of Scripting

Following through from Berne, the dilemma in a scripting process is how to maximise opportunity for love yet minimise the loss of love. This dilemma is born from the realisation that love is not unconditional, i.e., that people and the context make demands and that parents have needs, wants, motivations, and requirements from the infant. This takes me back to a key text referenced in Chapter Two: *Why Love Matters* (Gerhardt, 2004)—the instinct of the baby to reach out for contact and connection, alongside the lifetime of conditioning that is about to begin.

I think of script (Berne, 1972) as protecting alienated parts of the self from further damage. Simultaneously, by keeping these parts at bay, script contributes to the recesses of our soul. So, the scripting process is simultaneously creative and destructive. Script protects what can be salvaged yet acts as a kind of double agent because it buys into what is on offer in order to maintain relationship and connection with community. It is the negotiation an individual creates within a potential oppressive system. In using the word "negotiation" I aim to capture a sense of a process between an individual learning about their environment and the environment making demands for adaptation from the individual. It is not altogether easy to find the right sort of word as evidently learning how to fit into society is important, yet conforming is script bound. So, even using the word "negotiation" proves tricky, and from a radical perspective, could be part of the deception that we really do live in a free society where everyone is welcome. People need to survive in social groups, and it is inevitable that the norms of those groups offer the benchmark of what is welcome and accepted and what is rejected. With help from previous writers (for example, Fromm, 1956), I argue that rejection from the group stirs primitive terrors of not surviving because of not belonging. Hence, identities and self-expressions that are not validated or not welcomed can be internally rejected or repressed, alienated from the self and remain at risk of being lost, never to be recovered. Such components are outside of the script system. However, through decontamination and deconfusion, aspects of relational loss may find opportunities to be re-experienced. In meaningful developmental work and in psychotherapy, this process of self-alienation in order to belong and survive needs to be validated and understood. It is important that it is not simply pathologised without recognising the deep desire and need for people to belong, to survive in a group, and to present their more normative selves (see, for example, Minikin, 2021). Other writers have also captured their validation of this process. For example, Shadbolt writes, "It made perfect sense to me then that he should retreat somewhere beyond reach, an act of supreme sanity, in my view" (Shadbolt, 2012, p. 6).

So, whilst Sedgwick calls upon the benefits of frame of reference as expanding the notion of script, I tend to question whether our frame of reference is simply an expanded form of script, one that takes in the multiplicity of context, and how we negotiate our survival in it. To date, I am also aiming to blur the lines between health and ill health, script versus autonomy. Whilst I do believe that it is possible to expand our consciousness with each other, I am in agreement with Shadbolt (2012) when she writes:

> I have often been reminded in my work that when a client's situation, presentation, and decisions, however bizarre they might seem initially, are understood, the behavior, thoughts, and feelings that I might at first pathologise or think are self-defeating can be seen as the client's unique and creative way of managing the unmanageable.

> (p. 6)

Managing the unmanageable points again to loss and loneliness. Script has been and continues to be a useful way of understanding our narratives. Scripts are born from relationship within context and so thinking about them as unconscious narratives rather than as self-limiting pathologies seems so much more useful to me. It helps us truly hold more enquiry into the client's experience, it helps us understand how they have been alienated, and what it is that they need to grieve for. To my mind, this is radically more helpful than negotiating our work from the binary position of script (unhealthy) versus autonomy (pathway to health).

Awakening to Loss: "Open Your Eyes and Look Within"

In this section, I invite the reader to revisit Alan from Chapter Three. He came to me in a deeply distraught, confused, and desperate state. He had moved to my location from a major city as a result of new building work locally[1]. As a reminder, Alan was crying without understanding why and was frightened and overwhelmed with managing his feelings whilst still trying to function in social life. He was apologetic for his crying, embarrassed that it leapt out of him so. His crying could be thought of as an expression of Sullivan's "Bad Me". It caused him anxiety, threatened his sense of safety and security, and called into question whether he was a man that could function in this world. This version of "Bad Me" was part of Alan's self-system, his identification in script, and his sense that he was always less than as a man. His realisation that the dam holding his feelings back was not strong enough to keep such vulnerability at bay was initially devastating and causing him to feel overwhelmed and without resources to cope:

> The origin of the self system can be said to rest on the irrational character of culture, or more specifically society. Were it not for the

fact that a great many prescribed things have to be lived up to, in order that one shall maintain workable, profitable, satisfactory relations with his fellows … If the cultural prescriptions which characterize any particular society were better adapted to human life, the notions that have grown up about incorporating or introjecting a punitive, critical person would not have arisen.

(Sullivan, 1953, p. 168)

The quote from Sullivan calls into question whether Alan's crying was an expression of alienation or actually a bursting forward of sanity in an alienating context. His daughter had been born bringing new life and new vitality, as well as new demands, into his life. Her cries had seemed to evoke his own and he was seeking his way to where his overwhelmed state might encounter an experience that did not overwhelm the other. That was perhaps the hope.

At the time of seeing Alan, I did not consciously think like this. I was a relatively young practitioner, doing my best to understand him and his distress. However, looking back now, I realise I could relate to him and his social context even though our superficial social appearances seemed different. My three parental figures had known poverty. I too had experienced this during my childhood. I had been exposed to the challenges facing working people in this country. I could also relate to the sense of feeling confused and distressed without knowing why. Generally speaking, I was also a woman who could get along with men. As a growing girl, I had experienced some positive experiences of friendships with men and boys. During my adolescence, my mother and stepfather had mentored some working-class men—helped them to find new opportunities via education. My stepfather taught in higher education and my mother had studied hard in Nigeria to gain a degree so that she could enter a profession and provide for her three children. Their generosity and personal politics had provided background role modelling and reinforcement for some of the positive experiences I had of them in my life. The "normal" in my adolescence had been a kind of open house where prospective students with diverse identities and social, racial, and cultural backgrounds came and went, joined in with our family, and were generally welcome in our home. These encounters and connections with many of these young adults helped me to recover from some social anxiety and selective mutism that had been symptomatic of the more traumatic experiences of my earlier childhood. This open door was highly symbolic for me and was a potent force in pulling me from my more withdrawn and alienated self. I literally had to say "hello" to many people from many walks of life. This move to look out did perhaps save my life and opened up the possibility of finding myself in this accepting and more vibrant environment. My grandparents had all been poor and had died too young because of it. My parents, feeling the benefit of an education leading to a better life, were generous and wanted to offer help to others. It helped me witness a generosity in my mother, which is important to acknowledge. Through her and my stepfather I have been able to appreciate the privileges I have gained in life and have enjoyed the opportunity as a psychotherapist to also be generous.

Returning to Alan and his sense of his vulnerable self as "bad", we can see how this self-state has evolved out of what we have come to call misattunements in psychotherapy: "bad me ... is dependent, at this stage of life, on the observation, if misinterpretation, of the infant's behaviour, by someone who can induce anxiety" (Sullivan, 1953, p. 162).

Sullivan is referring to the developmental stage in an infant of 9–10 months, though I would like to propose a more ongoing process not dissimilar from Sedgwick's approach in that formative and deeply influential experiences don't just originate in the mother/infant dyad but from the holding environment (e.g., Winnicott's nursing triad), the family group, and the wider social, economic, and political context. If Sullivan is referring to an actual age, in terms of development, I draw from Mellor (1980) who also talked about ego ages. This is a useful way of thinking how situations that evoke deep hurt, pain, and trauma also create terrible anxiety within and this causes the vulnerable self, or aspects of our soul as I see it, to recede from consciousness—to be banished.

Alan had been getting on with his life. He had managed to establish a stable and loving relationship and he had always been ready for hard manual work, taking some pride in building a home for him and his wife. He was unprepared for the impact of becoming a father and the overwhelming experience of love alongside the vulnerability of a newborn infant had terrified him.

Oppression + Deception + Engagement = Awakening + Disturbance

When I first met Alan, I sensed I could see the man he was and feel the sort of life he led. I had an intuitive feel of him. My historical exposure and connection to working people must have been evoked and contributed to the non-conscious processes between us (Summers & Tudor, 2015). I think the pictures created by our historical and current life contexts offer a sense of connection and rapport which facilitate a working alliance. Alan described the stress of his daily work schedule and the enormous effort it took him to hold back his tears. The way in which Alan reported and revealed his process was very affecting for me. I felt both empathy and sympathy for his plight and I could vividly imagine his day-to-day struggles. These feelings and images stirred me to care for him, to feel warmth. We could think of it as a maternal and erotic countertransference which added some vitality in our encounters and contributes to the term "engagement" that

I am aiming to capture in my rewriting of the liberation formula. I wanted, and felt motivated, to get to know Alan some more. This atmosphere was a facilitative one and Alan was able to open up and share some of the stories from his childhood and earlier life. This built a picture of his life, some of which we would call script: a story that revealed the limitation of his aspirations and the way in which he had been oppressed, as described in Chapter Three. What helped him in talking with me about it was that explorative encounter of visiting and revisiting of the key themes in his story. This awakened him to the possibility that he had been missed, not only in his family but also at school, and in his early adult life too. Generally, he had received little encouragement, guidance, or role modelling that enabled him to feel valid and respected. Clearly, he had arrived to me already disturbed in confusing and distressing ways. The process of awakening and disturbance in Alan's story relates more to the deconstruction and reconsideration of perspectives from his earlier life. In Transactional Analysis we might think of this as decontamination, a kind of throwing light on how and why our internal worlds have become depressing places to inhabit.

Thinking about the way we formed our alliance, I understood that Alan was alienated from his feelings. And now, as a maturing man, they had leapt up and taken a hold of him. He was frightened about what that meant. It seemed to me that his crying was coming from a place that was "not him". Not a man. Not this man. So, the current state of alienation he seemed to be communicating to me was that he felt under assault from his feelings, and he was hoping perhaps I could make them stop.

And so, what did I make of his particular form of oppression and deception? I think it is the kind of damage that has been done for centuries to men here in the United Kingdom. It is a hard cultural stereotype to shift. It tells men, especially working men like Alan, that crying means weakness, and that crying is for women, not for men. That working men like Alan can at least hang on to their male pride by remaining strong. Tough. To lose their armour may feel somehow like losing their skin. Perhaps it feels like there may be nothing left to hold them together. This is a deception. A deception that Alan did not invent but that he has taken in, and so it is all the more remarkable that he came to see me.

Prior to seeing me, Alan had seen another therapist (a man) in the city he had previously lived in. Initially I had asked him whether he wanted to return to him, as it appeared he had appreciated seeing him and had found it helpful. He came to tell me how desperate he had felt every week and that this therapist had felt like a saviour to him. This made it all the more puzzling for me that he had not returned to him. When I asked him about that, Alan told me he had just dialled the numbers in the book, and I was the only one who actually answered. He had liked the sound of my voice. I never quite knew why he had decided to find someone new, or whether he had been actively looking for a woman. The impression I got was that having had a good experience before, in his state of feeling desperate, he simply launched himself into the local therapy community until he found a voice. The answering machines were not going to do it for him; he was searching around for someone who was alive, who answered him back. He just took a chance with me and was available to what I could offer him.

I drew on his previous connection and felt optimistic about the work we could do. In terms of his previous counsellor, it gave me hope that we would be able to go beyond his isolation, his alienation, and his terror that there was something fundamentally wrong with him. He had told me that he had a deep longing to connect.

Radical-Relational Reformation

As I remember those early sessions with Alan, I am reminded of how I was feeling full of him and his plight. Often my responses were simple empathic specifications, as well as some enquiries. I did not share the extent and depth of the feelings he had evoked in me. This was, I think, intuitive rather than informed by any particular training, technique, or skill set I had acquired. As I think of it now, I am reminded that at times of intense family difficulties, I often became a shock absorber in the family. As the elder child, I felt an instinctive need to protect my younger siblings and I think at times I needed to dissociate in order to do that. So, whilst I can often feel intensely for others, I am aware that my defences sometimes lend themselves to "stilling" my outward facial expression. This can at times give the impression that I am withholding. However, internally this experience can feel less about withholding and more about holding (Hargaden & Sills, 2002), which with someone like Alan was facilitative as the alliance developed. Becoming more aware of my tendency over the years and having been exposed to some psychoanalytical ways of working, I recognise that I was subconsciously striving to give an experience to Alan of space without too much intrusion from me. I think clients often need to feel a presence and engagement without a "colonising" of their mind (Chinnock & Minikin, 2015). I also recognise I don't always get this right, especially when under psychic pressure of the kind that happens when there is an enactment or strong feelings of projective identification (I say more about this in Chapter Nine). However, in the way that I have come to work, I see that initially I want to do nothing more than understand clients in the context in which they come. This understanding is about the beginning of their life in my mind.

In thinking again of Alan, I am reminded how I enjoyed his physical presence. The paradoxical presence of a strong body revealing vulnerability can be erotic for a woman like me. I am reminded that I appreciate the physicality of men, and this reminds me of my youth. As a growing girl and young woman, I had enjoyed sport, watching cricket in particular, as well as playing games and being outside. My appearance these days as a professional woman may not show this—for example, the hidden me that relishes physical work outdoors, especially in a garden. I said none of this as I sat there with Alan, yet such images and memories were in my mind. As he spoke, I was consciously, subconsciously, and possibly unconsciously connecting with what he said, building bridges that were the potential scaffolding for our work together.

I have spoken now of the earlier weeks with Alan, of how he may have felt some awakening and disturbance by our conversations. Yet a further disturbance was to come, not just for Alan, but for me too. As we continued to meet, his awakening as I understand it now, was his growing attachment to me and our meetings. He was sharing some mutual connections, some points of common interest, such as his love of gardening and the onions he grew that he was proud of. I did not disclose it, but he seemed to know I was a gardener too, and every so often he would check in with me about particular plants, or the chickens I kept, or what worked and what created mess outside. After nearly a year into the work, I had to tell him I was taking a long summer break. I did not reveal the reason, which was that I was getting married to my long-term partner, and we had planned a holiday abroad. On hearing the news of my break, Alan collapsed into tears. He and I were shocked by the impact. Fearing the potential for a breakdown, my supervisor advised me to make weekly contact with him over my honeymoon. It was a little challenging, as I was in a different time zone, but sure enough once a week we spoke on the telephone.

Reclamation: Awakening + Relational Connection

Playing with the idea that, fundamentally, psychotherapy is helping clients become more alive and vital, I think of the second phase of work as "reclamation" or "resurrection". I think both are relevant in the work, though in order to be clear about some of the differences, I confine my discussion of the work with Alan to considerations of what in him was reclaimed. This links to parts of the self that go into hiding, protected by script, so they are, so to speak, not exactly killed off, but decommissioned and sent into exile. I was drawing on the work of Stern (2010), Novak (2015), and Sullivan's (1953) "Bad Me" (or to my mind, "Banished Me") and "Not Me". In short, Sullivan named the parts of the self that cause anxiety because of the loss of love they evoke in the other ("Bad Me") and he also described parts that have been killed off or dissociated from. Stern described the enactments that erupt from dissociated parts, and Novak integrated these ideas into Transactional Analysis by clarifying the difference between games as repetition of past "Bad Me" relational dynamics and enactments as actions that are psychic material coming to life. So, as we become more alive to ourselves, new phenomena emerge that could lead to greater social and psychic flexibility with ourselves and others. I refer to such flexibility as the possibility of plurality:

Awakening in Self + Relational Connection Plurality with self and others

I understand that the shock for Alan and me was that on some level I had missed our developing bond. This is deeper than a working alliance and more of a feeling of belonging to each other. The strength of his feelings woke me up, disturbed me, and got me thinking more about bonding. The parallel in my private life was my move to marrying my partner; my partner who was "not Alan". So, returning from my honeymoon felt like the second key phase of our work.

On my return, Alan sobbed heart wrenching, deep cries. His whole body was shaking. I was stunned that he had missed coming so much, and it was a sharp reminder to me of the depths of his vulnerability and the impact of loss. I had gone away to be happy, to celebrate, and enjoy my time with my partner. I did not tell Alan that was why I went away, but he was feeling something profound about the loss of me. Perhaps he realised something about the limitations of our work, that we will not be lovers or even friends. Perhaps there was a reckoning that one day I will stop working with him, that we may never see each other again. His grief at that time was registering in my body, it was not just his, I felt it too. I was propelled away from the joy of my break and was back in the room. I registered how I had disturbed the rhythm of our sessions and that this had interrupted and cut him off from a sense of continuity, a level of familiarity and support that he had become used to. It was as if we both knew that in the fullness of time there was an ending that needed to be faced.

Reclamation: What Has Been Lost Cannot Be Reclaimed in Original Form

How do we transform what has been lost to us? Facing loss means there has been connection, belonging, or possibly love. There has been something to lose. Something was there; the loss feels devastating. So, thinking about Alan, I understand that he had lost the feeling of bonding. His alienation was caused by a breaking of a bond. The soulful part of him, the part that longed to connect had gone into hiding. I suggest this was a "Bad Me" identity because it had not been entirely killed off. He may have tried to banish his vulnerability but the part of him that longed for love, connection, and bonding was still there, and it was causing him pain. He was struggling to enjoy that part because the threat of that was too anxiety provoking. Anxiety that had been created to protect himself from the pain of such loss. It seems to me this was a case of mistaken identity. The part of him that he

110

was afraid of was actually the part that did long to connect, love, and risk bonding again. To help understand the sort of relational connection that helps parts to be befriended and reclaimed to some extent, I draw on Shadbolt (2012) and her thinking about the extended game formula.

From Games, Blame, and Shame to Shadbolt's "Extended Game Formula" (2012)

When Alan heard that I was taking a long break, he seemed to collapse, and I became very frightened. Some of my fear was valid in that intuitively I sensed the possibility of breakdown. The kind that would render him unable to function. The kind he was teetering on the edge of when he first came to see me. The eruption of Alan's vulnerability no doubt was a challenge to me and my scripting process around being important and having an impact. I had within my defences constructed effective ways to follow the path of least resistance and not cause disturbance to others, to not press upon them or demand of them. So, I was watching Alan fall over and that threatened my defensive wish to keep everyone and everything safe. Looking at this through the lens of classical game analysis could suggest that Alan presents himself in a vulnerable state and this hooks my defensive desire to soothe and calm in the pursuit of safety—a kind of smoothing over of distress. However, returning to Sedgwick's ideas that frame of reference is broader and wider than script, I also think that the history and my memories of relatedness that I described earlier in this chapter were also relevant. Hence, the defensive and the creative are held in tension together.

These moments of surprise or shock in the work, difficult though they may be, have come to be thought of differently in recent years. Shadbolt (2012) writes that,

> when ruptures and failures are cocreated between client and thera-
> pist, rather than being regarded as pathologies that stand in the way
> of the work, they can be engaged with as therapeutic change
> opportunities, their resolution being the central therapeutic task.
>
> (p. 6)

She goes on to say, "surprises can feel like attacks, and uncertainty can feel like failure, and both risk triggering the shame I mentioned earlier" (p. 11). Furthermore, Cornell and Landaiche (2006) foreshadow Shadbolt's position when they write, "disturbances seem an inevitable consequence of the intimacy that develops in every therapeutic and consulting relationship" (p. 197).

Despite my availability through my honeymoon, the practical, as well as symbolic, experience of this for me personally and professionally, recognised these telephone calls were inadequate. It is possible they may have kept Alan out of hospital, but on my return, he was shaking and fragmented as he described what he had suffered for the four weeks I was absent. In her article, Shadbolt goes on to say that there are no "specific techniques ... rather a set of relational attitudes and values ... All the therapist's experience, training, supervision, and personal therapy and his or her resulting expertise, wisdom, steadiness, and plain humanity are required at such times" (Shadbolt, 2012, p. 11).

As previously mentioned, I was a fairly young practitioner at this time, and I found Alan's overwhelming vulnerability catching. Unaccustomed to knowing I could have an impact on another in this way, I have since wondered whether on some level, Alan was coming to realise the limitations of our relationship: that we had connected, bonded in a way, but that was inevitably going to lead to a loss and the pain he already knew about surfaced again when I left him to marry another man. We never spoke directly about this because I have been and continue to be careful about what I disclose concerning my private life. However, it was important to process the experience and to find ways to help Alan with his feelings. Acknowledging the pain I had caused was a first step. Exploring the significance of the regular meetings and the rhythm this had created in Alan's weekly life was also important. There had been a felt sense of constancy and reliability as well as an interested, listening ear and someone that could relate to his emotional and vulnerable self without him feeling less of a man for it. Perhaps, on the contrary, he had picked up that I found his vulnerability along with his physical strength a source of attraction. I saw him as more manly, more human, and more loveable because he could reveal himself to me. Creating space to acknowledge these experiences, reflect back on them, relate them to his sense of masculinity and his identity as a man in the world, as a husband, and as a father was the important work we needed to do. Through this, he began to reclaim his vulnerability—not as an enemy or a threat to his manhood, but as a way more into it. Clearly our humanity is never going to be experienced in quite the same way as we did as infants, but some defensive behaviours and anxieties will inevitably live on. But it was a revelation to Alan and a new source of comfort that he could feel less frightened and more accepting of his feelings. As Shadbolt's extended game formula reveals, once a payoff (painful, often shaming, feeling) has been experienced, we are only halfway there. The next part—the reclamation as I am calling it—means that we need to acknowledge what has happened, and make space to explore and discover meanings that help us feel less alienated and more fully human and able to tolerate lives in our own skin.

Conclusion

There are many ways to capture the expansion of consciousness that clients experience from talking to a therapist. However, what does seem important to emphasise at this point are the nonconscious experiences of social and family context, of relations that create relatedness, as well as internal defensive processes that evoke retreat and shut down. The demands made that induce internal, interpersonal, and relational needs to close down or desire to open up can feel powerful. Cornell and Landaiche (2006) describe the interpersonal pressure from the client to the therapist and go on to stress that challenging encounters do not necessarily indicate the therapist is stuck in a pathological script bound process, "but is engaged in a level of experience with the client that is not yet available through words" (p. 199). This takes us from the experiences in this chapter that have focused on how to draw out and reclaim banished feelings and self-parts to the possibility of resurrection. How do we breathe life into processes that have been killed off?

Note

1 Across the United Kingdom there has been a policy to build as many houses as possible on account of a crisis in homing. A full social and political analysis of this endeavour is beyond the scope of this book. However, I imagine such an analysis would consider inequalities of wealth, multi-home ownership amongst the wealthy, the need to keep a capitalist system afloat (such as the housing market), and the environmental concerns such as increased removal of top soil, natural vegetation, and demands on infrastructure development.

9

WORKING WITH DISSOCIATION, ENACTMENTS, AND RE-ENACTMENTS

Introduction

In this chapter, I revisit the ideas I wrote about in Chapter Four which considered oppression and deception within a model of symbiosis. I proposed that when a more dominant object seeks to subjugate another, a gripping symbiosis can be established. This is possible when there is a lack of protection for the subject who may feel practically and/or psychologically compelled to consent to the oppression and continue to survive it because of being trapped in a state of dependency. I suggested such dynamics evoke deep states of pacification in the subject and I linked these dynamics to Bollas' idea of extractive introjection, which explains how resources get both undermined and taken, making systems of domination possible. These alienating processes inevitably feed into scripting and dissociation.

Dissociation and enactment have been described by a number of authors, (notably, Stern, 2010, and also Minikin, 2018, Novak, 2015, and Stuthridge, 2017). There are also links with Shaw's work on traumatic narcissism (Shaw, 2014). In his writing on games, enactments, and re-enactments, Novak (2015) distinguishes these different processes. He reminds us that games are repetitive transference dramas that are related to the scripting process. In other words, they are relational dynamics that are known to us, even though they may evoke painful experiences. On the other hand, enactments are expressions of unformulated experiences—dissociative processes that have not been known or developed within the self. They haven't had sufficient relational experiences to lead to a sense of cause and effect. And thirdly, Novak describes re-enactments as eruptions of past traumatic events. In other words, these have been known, but fiercely defended against via dissociation.

To illustrate, I return to the case of Emma from Chapter Four. Emma would sometimes argue with her husband about the support his sister got from his parents. Seeing the capacity of his parents to support her sister-in-law provoked feelings of jealousy, loss, and deficit within her for not having

DOI: 10.4324/9780429289231-11

had that kind of parental support. Emma knew this about herself and could talk about her feelings of frustration with me, telling me she did not like that part of herself who could feel resentful. The game, as I understood it, was the repetition of this fight with her husband who had to bear her complaints or react to them. The enactment between Emma and myself had something to do with Emma's capacity to offload to me and my inability at times to bear it consciously, hence my draw into sleep. Something was unformulated between us here and this experience needed to be reflected on, to take shape so that we could both take charge of our feelings so meaning could emerge. An example of re-enactment was the panic attacks Emma experienced. Here, her system went into overload when dysregulated terror erupted if one of her children became unwell. These were related to her childhood traumas of living with a father who was at risk of dying suddenly. I think these distinctions between games, enactments, and re-enactments are useful in helping to think about processes. They help the practitioner to organise their priorities about how to approach, respond to, and work with what is emerging in the work. The difficulty for me is that often such choice points are not so clear because there is often more than one dynamic happening at once. Furthermore, because the therapist could be compromised in the countertransference experience, this can make the whole co-created experience even more complex to navigate.

Dissociation and Trauma

Traditionally, dissociation has been associated with trauma and has been thought about as the overwhelming terror and helplessness that gets evoked through physical or psychic abuse or violence. Such events bring the subject or others close to them near to death, or fearing death. For example, I had a client who was traumatised because he fell down a hole on a building site. Luckily for him, he got trapped halfway down. Had he dropped right to the ground, he would have died or been physically disabled by the accident. This was not a relational event, but it became interpersonal and intersubjective when his unprocessed terror prevented him from sleeping or being free to play with his children. His children picked up on his terrible state of anxiety and they absorbed some of his deep feelings of helplessness. They also had their own frightened responses to the dysregulated introjection of feelings from their father. In a similar way, Emma had attuned to and absorbed her father's unprocessed terror. In addition, she experienced her own fear alongside his developing tyranny and aggression. Her hypochondria, inherited from him then passed down to her children, rather like Fanita English's hot potato (English, 1996). In other words, the experiences that have been too "hot" for parents to process get unconsciously passed down to their children. I suggest event-based trauma becomes relational trauma via proxy. This is particularly relevant for intergenerational and transgenerational trauma. Fragmented processes get passed on, meaning that dissociation arising from unformulated experiences may be associated with violent and life-threatening events, though the origins in the story have long since been lost.

A Personal Story

Many years before knowing about unformulated experiences, I arrived at my therapist's consulting room, to find the door locked. At that time, I was pretty much mute in my therapy, inexplicably unable to think or speak. I stood at the door frozen. I was at an utter loss about what to do. To ring the bell again or bang loudly on the door was unthinkable. To go away unannounced also had not yet come into my mind as a possibility. So, I stood. Feet cemented to the ground staring at the shut door. In a few minutes my therapist appeared, profusely apologetic and let me in. In the moment, it was as if I was utterly without feeling about the experience. Much as he invited me to say how it was for me, I could not. I simply did not know, or I could not let myself know. Somewhere I expect I felt unwanted and possibly imagined he would not want to see me given my inability to talk. I was a deadened mumbling client, and it was a long time before words came that could begin to put shape to that experience.

Today, I can think of the locked door and my frozen state as a game. For instance, I was repeating an experience from the past about an unavailable other and so diminishing my own emotional needs—to be as undemanding as possible, was one way of getting through life. The payoff being I could feel rejected or unwanted and the "unavailable/available" other could feel frustrated that for all their efforts to engage me, I could hardly respond. Alternatively, I could think of this experience as an enactment. Something was happening that was not yet close to being symbolised: the locked door and the frozen child. Perhaps it was an unconscious, dissociated experience that captured my felt sense of alienation? The alienating experience of having felt shut out or ostracised had developed an instinct in myself to shut down and shut out. This may have origins from the first few months of my life, when family circumstances kept me separated from my mother for prolonged periods of time. In addition, my dissociative responses could reflect the intergenerational trauma of other lost parents. My maternal grandmother was raised in a Victorian orphanage, for example. Also, could my capacity to freeze represent inherited trauma from my father and his witnessing of horrifying violence during the partition of India? In other words, being shut out of one's land or one's country. Fearing for your life because of who you were—your origins that you cannot help—you were simply born into them, and you find yourself unwanted, hated ... your very life threatened and your need to run to safety.

All of this could have been feeding into my capacity for profound projection and to freeze in the face of authority. In those few minutes, time had stood still ... My therapist's apology, even though I could not respond, did have an intense impact on me. It was the seed of something. The unexpected response to my presence as it seemed to suggest care. Thinking back, it strikes me that it is so important to take our time in these situations. I would have accepted the interpretation of this as a game. It would have confirmed the sense of myself as "Bad Me". I could have understood rationally that I needed to knock or ring the bell. That I could ask, check, and see which one of us might have made a mistake. However, such behavioural exploration could have meant that something essential about my being would get missed. I could simply assume responsibility for being inept in some way, feel ashamed and close down on the potential to discover what it was in my identity or history that was being re-experienced. Today, I am sure it had something to do with not belonging:

> The experience of belonging provides a vehicle for vitality, a sense of feeling alive with the possibility of an identity recognized by the group.
>
> (Morgan-Jones, 2010, p. 4)

It had been unthinkable that I might make a demand on someone I saw as deserving authority and respect. In addition, the possibility that this expressed something intergenerational, something that may have roots in event-based traumas was an important possibility and an insight to consider. In other words, when previous generations have had to shut down, or dissociate in response to overwhelming loss or violence, unless they get help with that, these fragmented experiences will get passed on to their children. Their children absorb them and also have their own responses making dissociation a most complex and multifaceted dynamic to experience and work with.

Dissociation, Thanatos, and Hypnos

My therapist once said to me that to read Shakespeare was the best way to read about psychotherapy. His comment caught my imagination, and I often went back and forth to one or two of my favourite plays and reminded myself of the wisdom and deep human understanding that was captured there. In Hamlet, (Act III, scene one)[1], Shakespeare reminds us that to sleep or to die is to keep away from pain, keep trauma at bay, and be temporarily cut off and unknown to our conscious minds. The desire is for comfort or perhaps the dream of a pain-free existence. In the same passage, Shakespeare states that the "body keeps the score" (Van der Kolk, 2015). Through my interest in working with dreams, I am also reminded that sleep cures, restores, and allows the body to rest and recuperate. To be deprived of sleep is a form of torture and to miss sleep affects our sense of being in and with health.

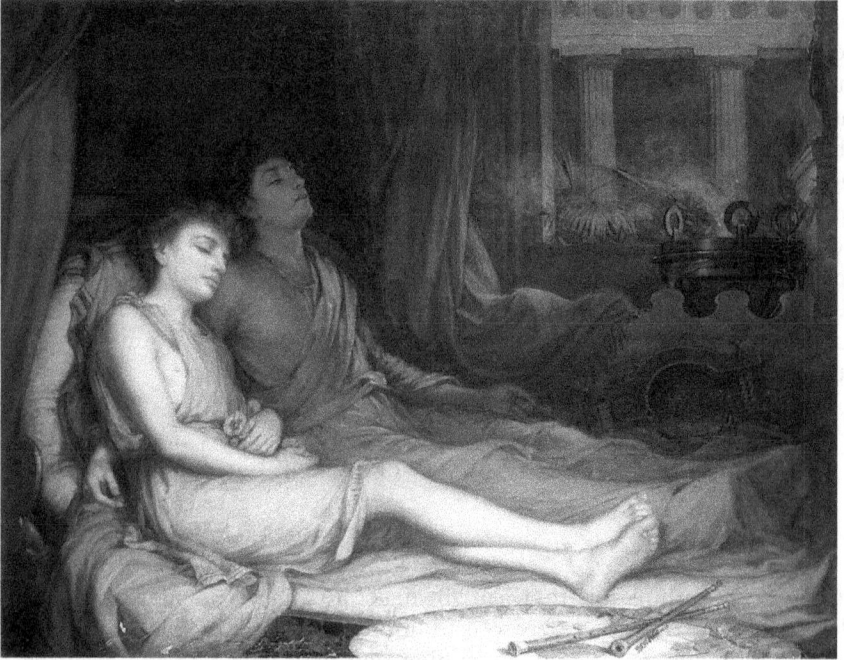

Figure 9.1 Sleep and his Half-brother Death (1874) by John William Waterhouse. (Image from Wikimedia Commons, file in the public domain.)

In Greek mythology, the twin brothers Thanatos and Hypnos represent "Sleep" (Hypnos) and "Death" (Thanatos). In 1874, John Waterhouse produced a remarkable painting of the two brothers sleeping side by side (see Figure 9.1). It seems to be an image of peace, contentment, and companionship. Shakespeare's words along with the image helped me feel more compassion towards myself for falling asleep with Emma. It helped me see another angle in my capacity to dissociate. It reminded me of the restorative function of sleep and the possibility of physical healing, and when dreaming is possible, the mind also begins to mend and seeks connections where experiences have been severed. To sink into sleep can be many things: a defence, an escape, a killing off, a surrender, a deep descent into the body and mind. Sleep is the reminder of a desire for peace.

Returning to Emma

So, in revisiting my capacity for sleep, I come back to Emma, from Chapter Four. As a reminder, Emma's father lived on the brink of death. From her reports, he sounded traumatised. He was volatile, quick to rage, and frightened, I imagined, and unable to face his vulnerability. He became a

118

controlling tyrant and Emma was terrorised by his tyranny. What he couldn't process, Emma absorbed, and so it seemed I caught something in relation to that when session after session I was pulled into sleep. I could grasp that I must be anaesthetising myself from something that felt unbearable. Emma pushed me to explore the pull towards death and sleep, and I was being challenged to find how I could move through such a powerful dissociative process.

Unlike the brothers, Hypnos and Thanatos, Emma and I did not sleep simultaneously. Rather, I slept whilst she chatted. When she first came to see me, she had recovered from a traumatic miscarriage, her father was living with her family, and she reported "walking on eggshells" around him. She was finding it difficult to cope and was hiding under her duvet and crying a lot. She was not sleeping at night and described getting up to compulsively clean the house. Presenting with an "overwhelmed" mind, she also described an overwhelming social situation clouded by uncertainty and her father's potential death. Since childhood, she had maintained her friendship with Daphne Ann, a Black woman of whom her father continued to fiercely disapprove. He prohibited visits by Daphne Ann to the house, even though he was actually living in Emma's home. Listening to Emma, I would relate to her by feeling overwhelmed by her life situation and distress. Although there are many aspects I could mention, I will limit myself to two key dynamics: Emma's sense of betrayal and guilt ("Bad Me") and her disso-ciated capacity to protest ("Not Me").

Mutuality + Engagement: Emma's Awakening ("Bad Me")

Earlier I described how Emma was oppressed and mystified by her father. Her childhood had the features of a traumatising narcissistic relational experience as described previously (Shaw, 2014). There were many examples of how she was subjugated to her father's mind. In the early days of our work, I understood she needed the support of another woman. In this sense, our social identities as "sisters" was an important source of relating. My listening to her story and responding with empathic transactions (Clark, 1991; Hargaden & Sills, 2002) offered Emma an experience that had been in short supply during her up-bringing. The difference in our race paralleled something important to her about her choice of friend. It supported aspects of her autonomy that were still alive. She was attempting to raise her family and cope with her traumatised father with a profound deficit in maternal input. Therefore, my capacity for empathy, relatedness, and connection to the sorts of oppression she had suf-fered were essential in helping her to build a more reflective, Adult ego state. As she did, she became aware of the depth of her guilt for betraying her father's wishes, and it was disturbing for her to recognise the betrayal she also felt towards her friend and then towards me for having inherited racism from him. Her attachment to her friend and, as the work progressed, to me were key in enabling her to challenge that state of mind. She literally became more awake to it, and she began building her resources. It was then, as I described earlier, that I started to become infused with sleep.

Emma: Awakening + Relational Connection ("Not Me")

The breadth and depth of Emma's psychological alienation included inter-connecting developmental, social, and other environmental traumas. A relational route to resolution had to come, in part, through my willingness to engage psychically as best as I could with multiple unconscious states of mind at work between us. Generally, unconscious communication and contact comes through transferential experiences, enactments, the imagination, and dreams. I think the strengthening awareness of both myself and Emma was crucial to beginning processes of liberation. However, reaching her "Not Me" state happened through a mutual experience whereby what was disappearing from our grasp needed to somehow be encountered in the clinical dyad.

At the time I started falling asleep, we had begun to speak about trauma. A recent need to visit the hospital had led to a panic attack for Emma, and we were reviewing her miscarriage with the terror, loss, and helplessness she had felt in response to her body failing her. Emma's graphic story of how she had miscarried raised horrifying vivid images in my mind and had triggered within memories of terrible, deep traumatic family experiences concerning birth and death. In addition, both Emma and I had experienced an overwhelming fear of death via the threat of losing a parent as a child. The absence of supportive women in Emma's childhood spoke personally to me too and contributed to my dissociative response of falling asleep. My awareness of shutting down, becoming passive, and not working evoked a "Bad Me" state, hence my fight against sleep to begin with. However, as I reflected in my supervision and personal therapy, I realised I was being pushed to engage with my impotency in the face of trauma.

After a few sessions, and drawing on reflections from supervision, I asked Emma about her relationship with anger. Initially, she stared at me blankly and did not know what to say. It was as if she had no connection to that emotion. To my dismay, my deadening sleep continued, so at some point I realised I had little option but to talk directly to her about what was happening, without knowing what might come of it. I declared to Emma that she might have noticed I had been falling asleep occasionally. She looked up and said she had wondered but had not been sure. I was curious to know what that had been like for her, and she said she did not quite understand what might be wrong with me.

It would be usual to expect a client to be angry that their therapist was falling asleep. It is not what we expect from our therapist—perhaps the last thing we come to therapy for. We might expect experiences of being betrayed, robbed, or discounted to emerge, especially if we were working

120

more directly with the interpersonal dynamics. Therefore, it was important to think about what might have been inhibiting her capacity to protest. How come she remained quiet about my disengagement? One of the parallels between her and myself and, then, myself and my therapist was the difference in class. I saw my therapist as being refined, cultured, educated, and more sophisticated in his knowledge and speech than me. Likewise, these differences were alive in my dyad with Emma, who saw me as the sophisticated one. So, it is important to acknowledge the power dynamic here: the perception of that and the capacity for that to affect the transference and countertransference in radical ways.

Returning to the ideas in Chapter Four, the less powerful client may trigger their spontaneous consent for the therapist to be in charge. The therapist's authority may go unquestionned. This is especially and ironically true when the client has formed a good alliance with them, trusts them, and believes they know what they are doing. In other words, the lines between ordinary respect and deference can become blurred. Should the therapist enjoy being appreciated or respected there is the risk of collusion, and the work becomes frozen or stuck. When I was the client, my therapist did not collapse, he was able to sustain his authority, and it was his kindness that mobilised me. When I was the therapist, I was initially unable to hold on to my vitality. Something about Emma's experience with trauma was triggering my own unformulated processes and hence the collusion was of a different sort. I was unconsciously abdicating from the situation. Had Emma been able to express anger or betrayal, I would have woken up for sure and we would have had something to get our teeth into. But she did not or could not. Just as I had not been able to protest standing at my therapist's door, likewise she could not. Something socially or psychologically must have been enormously inhibiting.

It had helped somewhat that our dyad had always had a social context that was spoken about openly. My home, my office, my language, and way of speaking revealed I had some education in my life and was living a middle-class life. Her life experience had been very different. We had previously explored the effect such differences in our social identity had on our working relationship. For example, her initial inhibition with me because of how I spoke was something we could draw on and work with. There were parallels she could speak of in terms of communicating with her children's teachers and school, as well as with some of the doctors she had struggled to talk with. We had both been willing to explore the impact of "othering" in our dynamic and my direct enquiries into the effects of race and class in our dyad as well as my history, which had included experiences of poverty, had created bridges. This meant that I couldn't quite be experienced by her as completely "other". Our intersubjective relatedness had also taken on a subtle quality, one that had navigated similarities and connectedness, as well as differences and disconnections explicitly and implicitly. Whilst this all sounds therapeutic, perhaps the subtle and unspoken elements between us had created a loyalty that also inhibited her capacity for straightforward anger when I fell asleep. To protest directly might have frightened her. This fear could be thought of transferentially as reflecting a fear she had with protest in her relationship with her father. It also reflects an inhibition that comes from wanting to maintain attachment to key figures—so, leaning towards toleration and forgiveness where there is some love. However, to collude with this also risked reinforcing the power dynamics between us, giving us scope to keep ourselves comfortable in pleasantness rather than delving into the discomfort—the shame I was feeling for sleeping and the feelings this needed to arouse in her.

Having raised the subject of my sleep, we began exploring this with associations to hospitals and the real, as well as metaphorical, death of a baby. Without saying everything in my mind, I said enough to let her know that this was something to which I related. I offered some explanation about overwhelming experiences, feelings too strong to hold. We also thought about her insomnia and explored projective identification, wondering whether I had been having the sleep for which Emma was desperate. Then we reflected on how impossible it felt for Emma to voice her objections to her father's racism and general tyranny. As we talked about her father, I was reminded that there had been occasions when I had wished him dead. My persecutory and rescuing fantasies had been evoked in the work, and I think of these as my connection with the rage I can feel in the face of tyranny. I consider this desire to be rid of the hated other as interesting; it reflects a capacity for resistance to oppression after all. However, if it goes unchecked, if it is met with unprocessed entitlement, it also reveals a capacity to inhabit a fascist state of mind—the very state I fear and wish to challenge in individuals, organisations, and the world at large.

As we talked, we drew, by contrast, Emma's attraction to Daphne Ann. Emma felt frozen with her father, yet her friend had been an irresistible choice. Emma had witnessed her friend fighting back at school. Back then, Daphne Ann had been defiant and raging, sometimes physically fighting the bullies who attempted racial abuse. Although this frightened Emma, her friend modelled resistance, which on some level must have had an impact on Emma. Although she dissociated from her own capacity, Emma was drawn to her friend, who could "do it". She watched Daphne Ann fight back and she served as a support for her friend, even though the fighting itself immobilised her. Daphne Ann became an important ally for Emma and, in my imagination, for me. As we talked about her, I recalled my attraction to strong Black women who protested. Memories of myself as a teenager, involved with the Anti-Nazi League of 1970s Britain and the associated fight against homophobia and the Rock Against Racism movement at the time, started to enliven my mind during sessions with Emma. I shared a little of those memories of earlier life in inner city Birmingham, an area inclusive of different races, cultures, and faiths in the United Kingdom. Emma seemed encouraged, and so began her conscious relationship with anger, rage, defiance, and protest. The connections between us and the image of Daphne Ann led to an awakening in both Emma and me that was furthered by our processing of the enactment.

Both Emma and I had the more typical role in the family of being peace builders rather than warmongers. Yet it was crucial that both of us could find the warrior and the fighter within to rouse us into a positive state of aggression and engagement with life outside and inside—hence my proposal for bridges to be built across social and psychic worlds. I think we needed to access our capacity to protest internally and externally. This points again to my proposal that the goal for resolution lies with plurality, which is found on the edges of what we reject or kill. Developing a capacity to tolerate and engage with different states of mind requires help from others socially as well as psychologically. These dynamics that push us to our edges yet also help us with them is what I mean by relational connection:

Awakening in Self + Relational Connection Plurality with Self and Others

The danger of totalitarian philosophies, thinking, and actions is that any relatedness with difference has to be killed off. It is as if to hear hurt being expressed is unbearable and intolerable to contemplate, and thus any shame or guilt within the oppressor also needs to be killed off or banished. To my mind, pluralism counters this position and offers a way forward towards greater acceptance within the self and with others as well as genuinely more creative solutions to social and psychological difficulties. However, I acknowledge the challenge therein. I died metaphorically and temporarily with Emma, and it was difficult and painful to move through this.

The theme of death and sleep is relevant for my second example here. And with this, I draw on a second literary author. The story I refer to makes a symbolic link between Emma and another client, who I call Colleen. Colleen is a Black woman, born in Jamaica, and she came to the UK to be raised by her grandmother when she was a ten-year-old child. My drowsiness with Colleen had helped me make some connections with the transgenerational trauma of slavery[2]. This is also the theme explored in complex detail in many of Toni Morrison's novels. Their exploration and portrayal of transgenerational trauma, gender politics, race dynamics, and much more are rich readings for all of us interested in the psychological fields. The story I refer to is from Morrison's novel, *Beloved*.

Reflections on Sleep and Transgenerational Trauma

In the story of *Beloved*, Amy Denver is a poor White woman who supports and helps a runaway pregnant slave, Sethe, the mother of Beloved. Amy and

Sethe meet in transit, travelling north—both searching and hoping for freedom. Amy helps by touching and treating Sethe's damaged feet and whipped back. She reassures Sethe that healing hurts (Morrison, 1988, p. 78). Amy goes on to deliver Sethe's child. It is a tender point in the book, evoking the connection that can be made between women in need. Amy literally has taken the role of doula and in so doing requests herself to be known too. She wants Sethe's child to know who brought her into this world. To tell her it was somebody. Somebody with a name, with a destination. It is a further cry of passion for bonding between women who are different, both have suffered, both known pain, yet able to help each other as they journey towards their different freedoms (Morrison, 1988, p. 85).

Morrison's writing, beautiful, painful, complex, evokes the challenges of class, sexual, racial, and gender trauma that lives on in many countries that have been involved in such historical trauma. She describes what is passed down through the generations. In one part, Sethe is relaying to another character, Paul, the passing of his mother. He can only know of this through her words, and he expresses his concern that his mother had suffered. Yet, Sethe reassured him that her death brough comfort, it seemed kind in comparison to what she had suffered whilst alive (Morrison, 1988, p. 7).

The actual and symbolic death of the mother has been a feature as a theme in psychotherapy: sometimes, in my view, without sufficient compassion for the context of mothering and the alienation that many mothers have experienced during their lives. This was the case for my Jamaican client, Colleen, whose mother was only fifteen when she was born. She had been a young teenager from a poor family who had a friendship and sexual relationship with a wealthier boy. Colleen's mother was still at school and so the extended family, especially her grandmother, was important in mitigating the overwhelming responsibility that can befall a young mother. I have been seeing Colleen for 25 years now and I have written about her previously (Minikin, 2011). What follows describes her story and the experience I had during the early years of working with her:

> Collen was referred by her doctor for depression following work-related stress provoked partly by explicit and implicit racism (Batts, 1982). She had also acquired diabetes complicated by self-neglect. Colleen's maternal grandmother had left Jamaica for England when Colleen was six and for the next five years different relatives looked after Colleen. Colleen described being passed from "pillar to post" across her extended family. And particularly in one setting, she had suffered physical and sexual abuse. Her grandmother in the UK came to hear of it and took action. When Colleen was eleven, her grandmother "sent for her" and she came to England.

In terms of my life experience, my connection with trauma had come during the six years of living in Nigeria during the Biafran war. The war and ongoing political unrest were present in the environs and was not uncommon in other African countries during those early years of independence. I had experienced West Africa directly as a child and Colleen carried something of this area in her ancestral unconscious. I had not experienced the degree of generational trauma and oppression that she had, although I had witnessed and identified with something nonetheless.

In our first session, Colleen asked about my racial and cultural background. She said it was important to her to see a person of colour. I asked whether she might prefer to see a Black therapist, but she said she would be ashamed to speak of her experiences and her life to a Black person. It was as if in seeing both my Whiteness and my colour she felt encouraged to speak about the racism she had experienced and later about the shame she felt as a Black woman and mother living in Britain. Colleen was married to a White British man and in recent years their relationship had turned deeply hostile. All of this added to the sense of alienation and isolation she was experiencing.

As Colleen started sharing her life, she told me of the effect of moving from London to the far north of Britain. In London there had been others like her—Black women married to White men. When she moved north, she was living in a White family in a predominately White community. She felt alone with a strong urge to hide. Most painful of all was hearing her regret the day she inflicted her Blackness on her children. Her naming this rekindled my history and memories of my shame regarding my colour and the violence and abuse I had been subjected to, particularly in childhood. I connected on some level to her sense of disempowerment as a young mother that could not protect her children, and this reminded me of my struggles in trying to protect my younger siblings at school. As I was remembering this, Colleen was reminiscing on her experiences as a younger mother:

Colleen: It was difficult for me to go myself to their school ... because of the possibility of my children not wanting to see me there ... as the Black half in the partnership ... whether they would—you know ... (looks down)

Karen: Feel ashamed?

Colleen: Quite often I wouldn't turn up and ... I've neglected a lot of their education because of that ... And the first time I saw my son at school with his friend, I was prepared to walk past him ... when he saw me and introduced me ... and that was the proudest moment of my life ... (crying)

Karen: So you wanted to protect your son from the shame he might feel for having a Black mother.

Colleen: (nods).

This and other similar stories moved me—the image of her almost walking past her son was alive, vibrant in my imagination. It reminded me of the generations of enforced separation and splitting of Black families through slavery and though this was different, it was a legacy of something important, something alienating—of not being able to claim your child as your own.

As I got to hear more similar stories, I noticed how my responses shifted. I sometimes felt disempowered and deadened in her presence. I would start to drift, losing connection with myself and with her in the process. Initially, my countertransference was difficult to make sense of, as on the face of it, Colleen was available for contact. However, over time I started to think of it as a shared sense of helplessness and dissociation connected to both personal and cultural trauma.

There was a paradoxical quality in Colleen that linked independence to deadening passivity. The experience was so profound—more than a one-generational scripting process, which suggested this was more than an individual adaptation and response to modelling from her grandmother. It seemed to hold an ironic flavour of enslavement. In other words, a capacity to Be Strong and survive by becoming deadened and impassive. I started to consider the possibility that the psychological process of slavery had been passed down through the generations via the maternal line. Independence was a façade and evidence of the deception created by the oppression of slavery. After hundreds of years, the trauma and oppression of slavery was evident in Colleen's presentation. Often, her voice would deaden, her face glazed over, her expression blank, and mirroring this, I would feel enormously drowsy.

Slavery and Gender Politics

As I referenced in chapter five, one of the most shocking texts that reveals the brutality of slavery is the speech attributed to the slave consultant of the eighteenth century, Willie Lynch. As a reminder:

"Keep the body and take the mind. In other words break the will to resist".

(Lynch, 1712, p. 24)

I had linked the transgenerational trauma of slavery in my work with Colleen. The experience of becoming sleepy with Colleen alerted me to the power of unconscious transmission in transgenerational trauma[3], and through this I was able to examine and make more sense of the dynamics I wrote about in Chapter Four. The conscious use of terror in order to control has left a social, political, and cultural legacy of almost global proportions. I still work with Colleen today, mainly to offer support. I only had some

126

elementary counselling skills when I first saw her, but that was not really the point. The point was she needed someone to relate to. Feeling alone, isolated, alienated from community, spouse, and the workplace, she was ready to take her life. It would have been easy for her as she explained it to me—she was diabetic, so she had the resources and the knowledge. She had been a nurse and was compelled to take early retirement as a result of an early stroke she had during her 40s. This had in part been a result of health complications from undiagnosed diabetes. Consequently, she was plagued with all sorts of physical challenges that were a struggle for me as a non-medical person to understand. No doubt I could write much more about her here too. However, suffice to say that it seemed important to her that I did track her bodily demise and need of help with it, as well as the demise of her vitality and will to live.

On Violence

According to Lynch, it was essential for women to witness violent and degrading acts. Emasculating the men in their presence and legitimising rape added to the apparent omnipotence of White men and was a further recipe for the psychological and physical traumas already experienced since capture:

> By her being left alone, unprotected, with the male image destroyed, the ordeal caused her to move from her psychological dependent state to a frozen independent state. In this frozen psychological state of independence, she will raise her male and female offspring in reversed roles ...
>
> (Lynch, 1712, p. 30)

This terror evoked a survival strategy amongst the women coercing them into meeting the needs of their White masters. To align needs according to those that oppress you is extreme and has been historically necessary. I believe such dynamics continue, albeit less obviously in some contemporary societies. These dynamics are also part of our transferential relationships in the therapeutic dyads, in supervision and in training establishments. I am not suggesting violent oppression is part of the process, but I am suggesting that where there is a power difference, there is always opportunity for oppression to be alive in the mix. So, although I could relate to Colleen and her capacity to freeze, her attachment to a kind of passive independence lured me into sleep. Possibly, it connected with my capacity to disconnect and to be devoid of relational relating. So, for all the warmth in our interpersonal relating, another dynamic was at work that was more deathly.

For Colleen, deeply held within herself there is likely to be what Morgan-Jones (2010) calls a primitive fear. He is drawing on the work of Bion (1961/2010) and Miller (1998) which describes a fear that exists in an individual or group in terms of not surviving because of not belonging. This fear results in individuals being driven to find ways they can survive and belong. For instance, the consent to oppression is a way of surviving, albeit at the expense of agency. In order for this state to persist, the person cannot grasp the full meaning of their self-sacrifice, so there has to be a disconnect from feelings. To have access to those feelings in an unprotected situation would be overwhelming and life threatening. Hence, oppressive "masters" are identified with and internalised, and that process gets turned in on the self, to perpetuate a state of being diminished and alienated from self-knowledge. This serves as the internalised oppression accompanying self-deception.

The work with Colleen reignited my historical and ongoing connection with people of African and Caribbean descent and also pushed me to revisit certain vulnerabilities in myself, such as my complex relationship with my race, gender, culture, life experience, and social and political values and how these manifested in my relationship or non-relationship with authority and aggression.

Both of the clients I have written about here pressured me to engage with a process at the edge of my capacity. I had the experience with both of having to struggle for life. And I couldn't do that by denying the death lurking inside me, the draw, the lure to sleep. I had to find some way through. The people that helped me here helped them too. Chains that enslave need to be broken and we also need to develop bonds between ourselves for reconnection.

Relational Trauma and Dissociation

Among numerous authors in the contemporary TA literature, Stuthridge (2006, 2012, 2015, 2017) has articulated a model grounded in an understanding of dissociation amongst states of the self and their emergence within the therapeutic relationship. For example:

> Integrating the fractured self requires an emotionally transformative process and often involves the unconscious participation of client and therapist in a series of shaky encounters. These collisions between two minds allow dissociated experience to be enacted, symbolized, and linked to a broader sense of "I." We discover "not-me" through an act of recognition ... feeling seen and felt in the eye of another.
>
> (Stuthridge, 2012, p. 239)

Traditional Transactional Analysis, as developed by Berne, was based on a model of repressive defences. The understanding of dissociative processes has extended the clinical reach of Transactional Analysis and is particularly relevant to the understanding and witnessing of the impact of oppression and alienation within the individual psyche and the therapeutic relationship.

128

Right at the start of this book, I stated that Transactional Analysis had radical roots—namely because Berne promoted a collaboration between therapist and patient and had a commitment to power sharing and taking joint responsibility in the work. Drawing on the relational principles that make use of relatedness through subjectivity and given the sort of radical Transactional Analysis that I am promoting, vulnerability is also mutual. Both therapist and patient face edges of consciousness and experiences that push at the edges of what is safe. As Bion (1961/2010) described, it was important for the therapist to also feel some anxiety as without that, curiosity is not alive. Hence, radical relational ways of working include the therapist being "radically open" (Hart, 2017) and therefore changed by her experiences with her patients.

Introduction to Chapter Ten

Whether we work as psychotherapists, counselors, educators, or consultants, we cannot escape the often unspoken fantasies and implications of what constitutes "normal."

(Cornell, 2018, p. 4)

It takes more than one author to write a book. Behind the scenes of this book have been my personal and professional collective. Deepak Dhananjaya is part of this group, and I wanted him to contribute a whole chapter because of his radical approach and work with marginalised communities in India. I have made use of context in this book, shown here as how we as individuals hold the collective through our families, our ancestors, and our social experiences. I have drawn on sociological perspectives to help widen an analytical gaze. Dhananjaya offers something critical here, something most important about reaching out to the ostracised, the "irrelevant" in society. Dhananjaya, like me, is trained in Transactional Analysis and is an important member of our international community. He is a grass roots therapist, a practitioner who is willing to go to the frontline and develop working alliances and soulful bonds with the forgotten people in society. In this chapter, Dhananjaya writes about his work with the women who help the invisible workers, the people who clean up after everyone else. I know there are others too doing similar work out there and changing lives through changing mindsets, and it is important to acknowledge that, and the very important work people are committed to.

In Chapter Ten, Dhananjaya writes about his work with the women who vouch for Dalit women. Western readers may have heard of "untouchables", and these are one of the most oppressed groups of people in the world. In addition to describing his work with this group of women, Dhananjaya shares his thoughts about alienation and liberation. He offers a critique of traditional ways of perceiving liberation, and he illustrates the way in which he stretches himself to work both radically and relationally with his own process. Dhananjaya describes how he confronts his own capacity to dominate, and his account reveals his deep humility and capacity for self-examination.

I am grateful to all those who have helped me with this project. It has served to develop my mind and my capacity for friendship and relationship generally. I hope as the reader finds Chapter Ten stimulating, humbling, and engaging.

Notes

1 To read the words to which I refer see Hamlet, Act III, scene I – his opening soliloquy.
2 See Minikin (2011) for a fuller version of Colleen's story.
3 For more on this, see Minikin (2011), or read the address claimed to be written by Willie Lynch (Lynch, 1712).

10

IS LIBERATION POSSIBLE? RADICALISING RELATIONAL PSYCHOTHERAPY AND COUNSELLING

Deepak Dhananjaya

The Kannada poem by Nisar Ahmed (1963) became a song that highlighted the way politicians herd people like sheep, enticing them to become compliant and obedient[1]. During election campaigns, the people are caught up, hypnotised by the personal goals of politicians, and so driven like herds of sheep! In this process, people pile up together and become one amongst others thereby losing individuality. This was an inspiring poem and song for me to think about the oppressive environment that is in India regarding religion, caste, sexual minorities, and the way social terror is created against them, inducing mob mentality. I see the mob mentality amongst mental health professionals who are driven by the definition of liberation defined by a set of privileged mental health theorists. I invite the reader to reflect on the idea of liberation throughout the chapter.

Introduction: From the Field to the Therapy Room

When I was eight years old, I was busy beheading ants as they moved in a line. At that moment, my grandmother got upset with me and explained that they feel pain, and that they are living beings. She emphasised that harming anyone who cannot fight back and have limited resources is unethical and inhumane. This incident and voice of my grandmother lived inside of me, and when I see any metaphorical beheading, I am reminded and I feel anger, despair, and hurt. This fuelled my journey of activism from the age of 16 onwards. I have been an activist for human rights, civic issues, and rescue operations of victims of human trafficking, etc.

When I turned 26, I was coming to terms with being gay in an oppressive culture, let down by my own religious beliefs and anchors, let down by a bureaucratic system of child care services, a victim of bullying and ostracisation by social peer groups, and having to deal with unrequited love. The activist in me got suppressed and I sought help to just be alive. This

DOI: 10.4324/9780429289231-12

experience led me to my own therapy and further inspired me to becoming a psychotherapist.

Psychotherapy training focused on developing a non-judgmental attitude, empathy, and unconditional positive regard based on Rogers (1959). This further suppressed the activist in me by fostering a compassionate, objective, and neutral view towards my clients and their issues. Unconditional positive regard and empathy were skills that I developed as part of my training and as a therapist. Eventually, I let go of my identity as an activist and became a psychotherapist. There were two self-parts of me, perhaps split: The Activist and the Therapist. These two parts were mutually exclusive and seemed unable to co-exist at the same time.

Therapist Turned Political

Being gay, I have lived an experience of exclusion and find myself in the margins in most communities and especially in my own country. Combined with my own life experience and working with different marginalised groups, I started realising that having unconditional positive regard and compassion with a neutral view or stance as a therapist was challenging. When I had to sit in front of a client who was a victim of institutionalised oppression with an "I'm OK/You're OK" belief, even if I truly did not believe that the oppressor was OK, was challenging. I believe holding a neutral stance would be like a bystander passively supporting the oppression. For example, it would be highly incongruent for me to hold a neutral view when a queer client discusses their stress due to a family's violence. I could not relate to the idea of having an "I'm OK/You're OK" attitude to the system or people that I considered oppressive. Holding this attitude comes from an assumption of equality in life situations for everyone. Minikin (2020) shares her view:

> For those with privilege in societies, all the time systematic oppression is sustained and functioning, there can be little incentive to labour with their minds long enough or hard enough to metabolise the collective traumas that continue through the generations. This is perhaps a reflection that those with more power in society are the groups that get to define 'OK-ness'—which then is bestowed upon or withheld from certain groups or behaviours. This is a socio-political perspective about power dynamics which has some differences from our liberal humanistic philosophy.

(p. 4)

So, continuing to hold a neutral stance in my work with clients seemed oppressive. In working with the marginalised sections of the society, I started to make a connection with their life situation to the oppressive nature of the political, constitutional, and social systems they are in. Knowing this, continuing to work with the intrapsychic process alone in order to help them attain autonomy (Berne, 1964) seemed limiting. I felt distress and the clients experienced a sense of being stuck. Clients come to us with some sense of "I am not good enough or not doing enough or I am unwell" beliefs about themselves. In continuing to work with a focus primarily on intrapsychic processes, the clients continue to feel "I am coming to therapy and still nothing is changing for me", then "I am not able to change, the problem is me!" or "I will never stop being unwell". This will reinforce the belief that they are the deficit.

This distressed me as a therapist and revived the activist in me, which has led me to develop as a socio-political psychotherapist. This process has helped me begin to find a way of integrating the two divided identities in me: Psychotherapist and Activist. My focus as a socio-political therapist is to look beyond the individual's intrapsychic processes and account for the socio-political context they are in, place the problems in the systems they are part of, and show how these influence the internal world and self-limiting beliefs of the client.

One of the ways I work with margins of the society in fighting the systemic oppression as a therapist is through psycho-education, staying with their social reality, and looking beyond the individual scripts of people to examine the external forces that often foster the script. This chapter describes some of my work with specific marginalised groups.

Liberation in Transactional Analysis

Berne (1964) said, "The attainment of autonomy is manifested by the release or recovery of three capacities: awareness, spontaneity and intimacy" (p. 158). He indicated that the individual is limited by the parental, societal, and cultural influences. Liberation from these influences is not an easy task, as they are deeply ingrained in the individuals. He affirmatively said that "individuals must attain personal and social control so that all the classes of behavior described in the Appendix, except perhaps dreams, become free choices subject only to his will" (p. 159). This essentially means that individuals have a choice of liberating themselves from their internalised parental, societal, and cultural messages. This liberation will help them attain autonomy. This will equip the individual to engage in "game"-free relationships. Traditionally, many Transactional Analysts have held and continue to hold this view while working with clients.

Although Transactional Analysis as a theory has evolved since Berne, TA as an application continues to exist in different forms; for example, the Redecision approach draws on Gestalt theory and methodology, working with different parts of self, early decisions, and redecisions. The relational approach holds a position that rupture in the primary relationship is at the core of distress

133

and working through that rupture in the therapeutic setting is the path to recovery. The important point to notice is that all Transactional Analysts work with interpersonal and intersubjective material of the client; their relationship with their mother, father, and other relational units (along with the socio-cultural influences). This interpersonal material along with the view of "Autonomy" as described by Berne encourages mental health professionals to believe that the individual can fight and overcome the internalised voices and oppression. Therefore, there is going to be a time during personal therapy for the client to choose to feel liberated. A liberation that may be an idealised illusion, given someone's economic and/or political conditions.

Autonomy as Liberation

The view presented by Berne of autonomy as liberation can be potentially oppressive when the individuals or the group are not limited by their internalised oppressive influences (parental, societal, and cultural) alone. Holding this view is oppressive when people are the victim of institutionalised oppression and are compelled to continue to exist in that oppressive environment. Institutionalised oppression is defined as "the systematic mistreatment of people within a social identity group, supported and enforced by the society and its institutions, solely based on the person's membership in the social identity group" (adapted from "Institutional Oppression", Tools for Diversity, TACS, 2006). The oppression can be hidden because it is so immersed in the culture of society and institutions. Nonetheless, it is also real for people in their current living environment. Some of the examples of institutionalised oppressions apparent in India are racism, shade-ism, caste and religion minorities, and gender and sexual minorities.

Steiner et al. (1975), as referenced previously in this book, provides a framework to begin to think about these situations. They argue that once people are angry, they establish contact with other like-minded and similarly experienced (oppressed) people. This awareness of oppression and coming together creates a social movement for change. The result of social movement can bring in liberation from the oppression. To remind the reader of one of the formulas:

Awareness + Contact = Action Liberation

I agree that within this framework, when people become aware of their oppression, may become angry with the oppressor. This expression of anger may invite collaboration with other like-minded people which may create a social movement. I think many activist movements can be explained to some extent by this formula.

I believe that this formula accounts for the contribution social oppression brings to the pain that oppressed people experience. This shifts the root cause of pain the oppressed community goes through from intrapsychic and script influence to social and environmental aspects. However, it operates from the belief that at some point the oppressed (collectively) can begin a movement and bring in change they desire, which in many cases is about respect and safety in existing within society—to believe at some point the oppressed will be able to make a difference is oppressive, if we have not accounted for the systemic flaws.

To illustrate this, I include an example of working with a psychoeducational group with therapeutic intent.

Group demography

The group consists of 20 women who are from a marginalised section of the society in terms of caste (Dalit).

Dirks (1989) explains that the caste system provides a hierarchy of social roles that hold an inherent characteristic and, more importantly, remain stable throughout life. The hierarchy influences the segregation of people based on caste into dominant and non-dominant castes, the food culture of the group, endogamy, and social meanings to the caste: pure as well as impure. The caste system also determines the type of occupation one is allowed to engage with. Macroaggressions like untouchability, denial of access to water and temples, are prevalent in rural areas of India, and microaggressions continue to exist in many parts of urban India too.

I quote this description from the Minority rights website:

> The term Dalit means 'oppressed', 'broken' or 'crushed' to the extent of losing original identity. However, this name has been adopted by the people otherwise referred to as Harijans, or 'Untouchables', and has come to symbolize for them a movement for change and for the eradication of the centuries-old oppression under the caste system. In legal and constitutional terms, Dalits are known in India as scheduled castes. There are currently some 166.6 million Dalits in India. The constitution requires the government to define a list or schedule of the lowest castes in need of compensatory programmes. These scheduled castes include converts to Sikhism but exclude converts to Christianity and Islam; the groups that are excluded and continue to be treated as untouchables probably constitute another 2 per cent of the population.
> (Minority Rights Group International, 2008, para. 1)

Dalit caste is a scheduled caste in the Indian caste system and finds itself in the lowest category in the hierarchy of the caste. Dalits (people who belong to this caste are commonly called this) are treated as "untouchables", although its constitutionally illegal to discriminate. There are private activist organisations that work for the rights of the Dalit community. This group of women work for the rights of Dalit women, especially when they are faced with caste-based violence (physical, sexual, psychological abuse). They work in the field with many stakeholders to fight for the rights of victims starting from advocacy, formal complaints with the police authorities, educating the families with procedural information, compensation for the victim, rehabilitation of the victim, etc. This is important background information to keep in our frame of reference, as the group of 20 women are well-informed activists who face society and legal authorities with potency.

The objective of the work

The objective over nine days with this group was to equip them with mental health awareness and basic counselling skills. The initial plan was to offer resources with skills building (counselling and introduction to Transactional Analysis). As I began introducing the topics, they were in touch with their own life experiences. This process quickly turned into a support group discussion along with the skill-building module. This meant that when I was teaching structural ego states (Parent, Adult, and Child) and the intrapsychic process, the group members were getting in touch with their own ego state content. In this process, they were able to see how their internal Parental messages were oppressive because they were women. They started sharing how they feel they are constantly trying to be a "good mother/wife/daughter/sister, etc." and these are all expectations of society. There were two processes in play at that time: one was that they felt safe to share experiences from their personal lives in the large group; the second was that they were identifying with each other's pain (of oppression). It was intriguing for me to see that these women who work for human rights of a particular kind of oppression (caste-based) were also having difficulty in recognising their own experience of being oppressed as women. As they were sharing, they experienced a process of mutual respect, a feeling of equality, of being heard without discrimination or being patronised or victimised by each other and me—a sense of camaraderie. I kept my focus on confronting the internalised patriarchal oppression and their ideas of being a "good mother/daughter/sister/wife, etc.". As for myself, being a cis-gender man in a patriarchal society confronting the patriarchy was different than what they were used to and it was impactful for the group, and helped the group build trust and alliance with me.

This was an experience of catharsis for the group. Cathartic as it was, it also helped the group drop into Child ego state (Berne, 1961). This seemed to evoke a collective Child ego state of the group, which was feeling heard and empathised with by me, as I was using many empathic transactions, especially empathic specifications (Hargaden & Sills, 2002). To clarify, this was not a formal therapy group, rather it was a bridge between a psychoeducation group that experienced a therapeutic component. In terms of the content of our discussions, I was imparting knowledge on Transactional Analysis and counselling skills. In terms of process, there was a relational experience between the group and myself. Since the group was experiencing me as different from other men of similar profile, and was building trust, I also had a counter-transferential (a sense of feeling good and a narcissistic high) response to them. I noticed I was feeling omnipotent, and the group felt compliant towards me. As a socio-political-relational practitioner, it is important to explore this experience. Rather than judging myself or the group, as I was becoming aware of the "Teacher–Student" dynamics in our system which has a legacy of submission of self to teacher (guru–shishya), I considered our multiple identities and invited the group to do the same. For example, I am a cis-gender gay man, from a more dominant caste, living in a metro city, and an English-speaking teacher. The group predominantly were non-English speaking students, from the rural parts of India, and mostly Dalit, cis-gender women. The generalised intersection of these multiple identities between myself and the group gave rise to a dynamic that encouraged compliance. I can understand this through interpersonal intersectionality (Dhananjaya, 2022) between multiple identities of the group and myself, so that the dynamics of our privileges and deprivations reinforce a normative way of relating. Hence my interaction (with respect) with them was a powerful confrontation to this dynamic and was countering their previous experiences of interacting with a dominant caste, urban-bred, cis-gendered man. I make this point explicit as this group of women encounter oppressive attitudes of men who are in the police department, bureaucratic services, and in their family and social environment (who have similar identities as mine) in their daily interaction. The patriarchal environment around them constantly reinforces their internalised oppression, and it is a *radical, rather liberating change* for them to experience a man (holding many different identities) to be different rather than oppressive. This helped the group to feel safe.

Despite my intention for egalitarian dialogue, I was aware of my potential dominance, so I made a more political statement to the group "We are a collateral damage of the societies' flaws". This came during a discussion about the microaggressions that women face in the current situation in urban areas, especially Dalit women. Even in metro cities, the caste of women is identified by their last names as well as through the dress they are supposed to wear. Many situations are oppressive towards women in general; however, there are further intersectional challenges from them being Dalit women.

This statement was a crossed transaction between myself and the group, as the group was expecting me to reinforce societal oppression. After I said this, there was silence in the group, as if they were not able to comprehend or were in shock to see a "cis"-gender, privileged, dominant caste man speaking out on such a subject. I held an important power position in relation to them and I was naming it. Most often the privileged section of society does not hold respect (consciously and unconsciously) for the Dalit community and even so for Dalit women, and so there was a puzzled expression on their faces and one of them asked the other group member, "Is it true? Like are we collateral damage of the society's flaws?" The question came from this group despite their awareness of legal rights, working in the area of rescue. They are activists who have been fighting against oppression (against caste-based atrocities). Holding their surprise (amusement) alongside their activist identity was revealing the mystification of oppression (against women) in that group for me. This awakening of internalised oppression highlighted how microaggressions work to keep norms in place that they experience every day as women.

As the conversation progressed, there was a process of realisation, or decontamination (Berne, 1961), that the flaws are not necessarily in them as Dalit women, but in the way the society has framed them. This helped in raising the collective consciousness of the group. There was relief and a feeling of liberation in that moment within the group. There was also a rising of collective anger towards society's oppressive frame towards them as Dalit women. I believed that this was valuable intervention for the group and would result in some form of action that could lead to a version of liberation.

What Next? Did It Lead to Any Version of Liberation?

This question confronted me, and so I explore it in this section with you, the reader. The group still has to go back to the oppressive society and face the macro and micro aggressions. Can they hold a sense of freedom? If so, how could this sense of liberation be compared to the way a dominant caste section of the society experiences feeling free? Because the women came together, can this collaboration affect society around them and support or tolerate their sense of liberation?

Steiner et al.'s (1975) formula added a few stopgaps to Berne's idea of autonomy, yet still ends with the idea that once the social movement has started, the liberation from the oppression is a possibility. To my mind, this formula still misses the idea of accounting for the current environment of the individual/group and its ongoing oppressive nature. It also misses accounting for the consequences the individual/group can face for their anger and social movement. Experiencing resistance from the mainstream, the group might feel incompetent and feel they cannot fight back against such opposition and so sink back into finding deficit in themselves even after the sense of liberation. Despite this, it does not mean that there is no value in the original liberation formula.

Further exploration is to understand the complexity of social pressures as a mental health professional who advocates the liberation formula yet also has to account for the consequences of teaching it, and exploring the meaning of liberation in itself. This formula helps in fighting the internalised ongoing oppression and realises that the core of the problem is within society and not individuals. This helps the individual and group to cathect their vitality, their physis (collective physis) (Berne, 1961), thereby feeling internally liberated and coming to know that feeling perhaps for the first time.

In my view, there needs to be an addition to the formula that accounts for the real and current situation of the environment that the individual/group belongs to. With this comes awareness to explore the safety of the individual/group if they retaliate against the oppressor. Do they have resources to face the consequences? How will they cope with the oppressor, who is not going to change or is a majority autocratic group, or society at large?

The danger of not exploring these aspects is a naivety in that the individual/group may feel internally liberated and have unprotected failed attempts at challenging the oppressor. This may lead to a reinforcing of oppression—one via the hand of the oppressor, another set up by the mental health professional who consciously or unconsciously is saying, "you have the awareness of the oppression, you have come together, and now you should be able to make a change towards liberation by fighting the oppressor". Given the reality of power dynamics, this could reinforce a sense of victimhood and inadequacy in the group. Thereby immobilising the group as they encounter a potential threat to their survival by trying to fight. Cornell (2018) states:

> For real change to occur, we must acknowledge within ourselves the depth of our not-OK beliefs and attitudes toward those who are different from us, whom we see as threatening, dirty, malignant. For real change to occur, we must expose ourselves as individuals and within our familiar social groups to those who hold us in not-OK positions and whom we hold in not-OK positions. We must be willing to engage with our personal ignorance and bias. We must place ourselves in circumstances within which we are confronted by others about our own ugly biases and projections. More than anything else, real change comes through our active engagement in the real world doing things.
>
> (p. 12)

And I do strongly believe it's important for us to hold his appeal while we work with the marginalised minority groups.

As we develop a radical psychiatry frame, it is important to expand the process and meaning of "liberation". I suggest:

Liberation = internal liberation + function of accounting (external environment, agency to tolerate consequences) + recognition (recognise the reality of futility and choices)

Along with internal liberation (based on Steiner's formula), it is important to account for the external environment of the client, their agency to tolerate the consequences of retaliation, and for all parties to hold recognition for the choices the client may make given the possible futility of their situation.

In the example I have shared, the group felt a sense of liberation as an experience of their work with me. I continued to work with them to understand the ways they would contextualise this feeling of liberation and account for the real society which is still oppressive. When they account for this reality, they may choose to challenge the societal norms in a few situations where they can tolerate the consequences, and in other places they may comply and give into oppression with awareness, rather than adaptation or quiescence. This part of the workshop was useful for them, as they felt I really understood them and was walking alongside them with the real and very repetitive oppressive challenges they live with every day of their lives. They experienced a sense of empathy for themselves knowing the choices they might make, which could include compliance to the oppressor. So, it provided a sense of greater stability for the group.

Socio-Political Therapist in the Room

Hanisch (1969) comments on the word "therapy" as "the very word therapy is a misnomer if carried to its logical conclusion. Therapy assumes that someone is sick, and that there is a cure e.g., a personal solution" (para. 2). In this regard, when a client comes to therapy, especially from marginalised sections of society (women from a minority caste or religion, a gay client in a society like India, etc.), the therapists look for things that need healing or curing in the client. As psychotherapists, the frame moved from "what's wrong in the client" to "what's going wrong for the client". DeYoung (2015) explains how relational psychotherapy is different from other forms of therapy. However, this work is still in the realm of looking at relational units in the client that get evoked interpersonally and intersubjectively. In thinking like this, we use our countertransferential experience to explore the therapeutic relationship dynamics that emerge and make a connection to a client's issues and work through them. As relational therapists we offer an authentic relationship for the client to process their grief, hurt, and anger that emerges between us (therapist and the client).

As socio-political therapists, it is important to expand our view from "what's going wrong for the client?" to "what's going wrong for the client due to the socio-political-cultural system they are in?" In this we don't just explore our countertransferential responses with the lens of "why do I feel the way I feel with this client and what is the client trying to unconsciously communicate to me?" We explore the countertransferential experience with the lens of "interpersonal intersectionality" (Dhananjaya, 2022). As I have written earlier:

> The individual's pluralistic self exists not only intrapsychically but also comes alive in its interaction with society (other people). When more than one person come together, they do so with their pluralistic selves. The power dynamics that emerge between the people involved are like multiple identities (pluralistic selves) of each person interacting and negotiating with multiple identities of another person … This negotiation is unconscious and unaware for each of us if we do not pay attention. Social and political therapists keep any power dynamics that might emerge between the multiple identities of both client and therapist as a major focus in the therapy.

The relational approach in Transactional Analysis, which is based on a two-person psychology (Stark, 1999), provides a model for exploring the dynamics just mentioned. Exploring our countertransferential responses to the client is important. When we experience anger, power, guilt, shame, pleasure, excitement, and so on in the relationship with a client, there is often a tendency to make it about that person. Clients do evoke such responses in therapists, and it is important not to reduce them just to understanding the client and their world. It is crucial to also explore the intersection of multiple identities that are interacting interpersonally with the client. This will likely lead to becoming aware of the systemic oppression at play between the therapist and the client (Dhananjaya, 2022, pp. 8–9).

I illustrate this with another example.

A client of mine (a woman) is in an abusive marriage dominated by a dynamic of coercive control. They have two children (three- and six-years-old). She is 35 years old. In my six months of work with her, we have addressed the internalised influences of parents, religion, society, etc. Initially she felt that she was an improper mother and wife, and hence the abuse by the husband was justified. Through our work, we unpacked her beliefs about being a woman, wife, and mother and the oppressive impact on her. She realised that she was collateral of the patriarchal system. She was in touch with her anger. Then she started speaking about her experience with her friends and realised they were also going through similar experiences as women. This connected them together. So far, the Steiner formula of liberation works well. However, the environment in the here and now is unchanged, and she is still driven by a patriarchal system.

At this point, if she retaliates or challenges her husband and in-laws, there are going to be consequences. To believe that this awareness and sense of camaraderie is sufficient to help her make the change could be dangerous. She is financially insecure and depends on her husband's income. She lacks support from her parent's family as they also live by the same patriarchal structure of society. She is not in a state to end the marriage as it can be unsafe for her existence. If I hold a view that with this awareness and psychological, moral support from therapy and friends, she can make the change, then whether I state it or not, she will feel like I am disapproving of her decision to stay in the marriage despite the abuse. This will add to the here-and-now oppression she is already facing, since she gets caught up in a dilemma of which man to please (husband or therapist). It may potentially reinforce her inadequacy: "I am not strong enough to quit this relationship despite the support I have". This is not helpful for the client.

In this example are identities of gender, sexuality, and economic status identities interacting with each other. This exploration helps in understanding the systemic oppression of the situation of the client and working through it without getting caught in the power plays or holding a neutral or indifferent view of the client's situation. As a socio-political therapist, it was important to explore my countertransference experience of frustration with a socio-political lens. In containing my feelings for wishing she could have a better life, we could examine the current circumstances for the client—their life situation and the social and political situation for them, rather than seeing her response to her situation through a pathological lens. The pathological lens often goes something like this: "This experience of frustration tells me something about the client's stuckness and/or her historical experiences". Whilst there may be a reality to the historical material of the client's life, one cannot discount the current situation the client lives in.

I held this in mind while working with this client and she was able to feel deeply understood and empathised with. This seemed to help her feel empowered and able to think about her life. She took small steps towards saving up, upskilling herself, finding a job, negotiating with the family, dealing with the societal shame towards her, before finally quitting the relationship. This happened over a period of two years.

Radicalising Relational Psychotherapy

From my experience of working as a relational psychotherapist and developing a radical lens (my socio-political view), I offer two qualities that are required for therapists to work this way. They are:

1   **Tolerating the futility**: As therapists, we intend to provide a space for the client to reform. Many times, during my own supervisions and my supervisions with my supervisees, it's easy to attach our value as therapists to the change our clients make. This has a sense of narcissistic

gratification which can be an unconscious phenomenon. Hence, when we see clients stuck in an oppressive situation, and they are in therapy, we want them to change and move towards a freer life. I think it is important to detach our value as therapists from the change our clients make. It is also important to tolerate the futility in their situation and the choices they do make. The futility could reflect the continued oppressive situation in their life, their lack of sufficient resources to move out of that situation, as well as possible internal resistance and fear of not surviving. This ability to tolerate futility will help in taking time to reflect on the socio-political lens.

2   **Advocacy**: As therapists, we are engaging with our own internalised oppression and our clients' internalised oppression. It is important to counter this internalised oppression with information and to be a potent advocate for the oppressed. This may be disapproved of therapeutic practices; however, I believe it's important to be informed and provide that information to the clients to counter the oppression from Parent ego states (Berne, 1961). This can lead to decontamination (Berne, 1961), as illustrated in the group case work.

What Is the Risk of This Perspective?

The potential risk of holding the lens of a socio-political system alone and placing the deficit in the system is that it can foster victimhood. We, as therapists, continue to work with the intrapsychic process of the clients. Simultaneously, we look beyond the client's intrapsychic process and explore the possible socio-political influences on their life and mind. In my opinion, we continue to help the clients realise their potential within the system they are in and help them navigate their challenges within those constraints.

Re-Thinking "Mental Health"

When we start thinking of mental health, we often hold a conscious or unconscious reference to physical health. Hence, we go to doctors when our physical health is upset, and we go to therapists when our mental health is upset. This means that there is something pathological which needs diagnosis and treatment. Hence, our theories and the literature are focused on finding the source of pathology.

In my opinion I strongly believe we need to rethink the way we understand mental health, and our job as mental health professionals. Mental health is not about wellness. Mental health of an individual is a reflection of the individual's context and environmental factors, such as food, security, safety (physical and psychological), and acceptance, as defined by Maslow (1943). Our job as mental health professionals and even so as socio-political therapists is to develop a capacity in self, individuals, and the communities to challenge the overt or introjected oppression and help develop a voice of their own! In doing so, we will cure the society of its oppressive ideologies and systemic oppression, because sickness is not in the individuals alone, rather they are symptomatic of society. This means our job does not end in the therapy room, it starts in our everyday interaction with the people around us!

Conclusion: Liberation—Reality or Myth?

When you feel you are stuck and not making progress with the client, it might help to reflect on the impact and influence of the system in which the client exists. Do they have a choice? How much of your thinking is based on the privilege of being a therapist? What is the client hoping for from you? What change are you consciously or subconsciously hoping for in this client? Is liberation a realty or a myth? In exploring this, you may encounter the futility, or limitation of their possibilities.

There is a thin line between advocacy, activism, relational therapy, and radical psychiatry. This work is an attempt to weave something together to be inclusive of the current life circumstances, along with the early ruptures, of the client. In this endeavour, I have made use of the combination of psycho-education (as explained in the group example) to provide information to counter the Parent ego state (Berne, 1961), tune to the client's early ruptures, and provide a stable other within a professionally contained authentic relationship, amongst many other therapeutic tasks.

As I reflect on this chapter, I wonder if "liberation", "autonomy", "cure", "change", and "transformation" are social constructs created by privileged mental health professionals from their lens of social safety. There is value in these ideas, and yet swallowing these ideas whole without deconstruction can reinforce the oppression of social situations. I hope that as mental health professionals we can make use of our life experiences, including our privileges, oppression, pain of alienation, and isolation. This could lead to greater attunement (Erskine, 1993) of our clients and ourselves. Attunement is towards the social context and oppressive elements in the ecosystem of ourselves and the clients.

For me, it is familiar territory to navigate as a mental health practitioner or as an activist; however, as I develop my identity as a socio-political therapist, I am caught in unknown territories. I am constantly confronted with the ethics defined by the mental health profession and the role of an activist, and I tread this path with careful consideration, self-doubt, peer conversations, and supervision with practitioners who are similarly oriented. In this process, I often ponder on the questions such as "Who is the guardian of ethics? Who says what is right and wrong? Or ethical or unethical? Or who is a good enough activist or not?" I realise these are my internalised ideas introjected from both communities to which I belong (mental health and activism). I appeal to the reader to join me in the process of expanding our territories of boundaries so we can show up to our clients inclusively—as these boundaries are not tight compartments! If not, we are in danger of becoming a muted, complacent herd of sheep introjecting the oppressive ideas of mental health!

Note

1 The song from the poem can be heard here: https://www.youtube.com/watch?v=5gYDp8PerSc.

11

THE RELATIONAL-RADICAL AND THE RADICAL-RELATIONAL

Recently, I was delivering some teaching on power, authority, and responsibility and I was asked, "what do I think is the greatest social injustice?" This was an interesting and unexpected question for me. It was asked at the beginning of the teaching day, as part of an exercise I do in inviting the group to get to know me and vice versa. My intuitive response was "inequality of wealth", and it was hard for me to think or move beyond this. I couldn't be drawn into a debate of injustice hierarchy, and I realised as I processed my gut response that I truly believed this was at the root of things. That, in order to fix the climate crisis and wider social injustices, the oppressed need to have more power, more influence, and more share of the wealth. However, the wealthy are not about to relinquish their assets—it takes tenacious effort to persuade the powerful to share their power. This seems to be the case at systemic, institutional, interpersonal, and individual levels. It has become hard to share what we have—except when our humanity is touched: when we love, when we feel compassion, when we respect others, and feel a sense of togetherness and trust. We have seen people inspired to be generous during times of hardship in recent years, and it seems that being generous and kind can be good for us, good for our self-esteem, good for our sense of well-being and feelings of satisfaction in our lives. So, as I come to the end of the book, I remind myself that we and our nations continue to be a work in progress:

> Somehow we've weathered and witnessed a nation that isn't broken,
> but simply unfinished.
> > (Amanda Gorman, Joe Biden inauguration speech.)

In the previous chapter, Dhananjaya explored the dynamics between the relational and the radical. He critiqued how we think and work in the psychological fields, how we account for inequality of power and the reality of prejudice, and the macro- and microaggressions that are a part of everyday life for some people. He explored our therapeutic frames, putting relevant and significant questions to the readers and writers here. This

DOI: 10.4324/9780429289231-13

concluding chapter picks up on the play between the radical and the relational. As I have been exploring since the start of this book—how do we engage the radical with the relational and the relational with the radical?[1] In my practice and teaching, I have been making a case for their mutual influencing in the movement between internal and external deconstructions of self and the collective. I trust that through the course of the book, the reader has also experienced something like this. The relational approach has helped me expand and deepen my work by the necessity of self-examination. The radical approach helped me investigate the dynamics of my intersectional identities, life experiences and think about these in relation to clinical, supervisory, and teaching experiences. It allowed greater scope to make use of who I am. Personally speaking, the radical and relational boundaries for me have not been separate entities. In terms of the academics of the approaches, the relational has included social and cultural implications, but has generally emphasised the significance of early attachment and attunement with the main carer, usually given to mean the mother. The impact of the social reality and the role of politics, economics, and social and cultural factors have been minimised, and the outcome in my view is further oppression of the mothering role, often held by women. The radical did account for the system and how this oppressed the vitality in people, misused resources, and deceived people of the meanings in their life. The analysis of the outside was taken seriously. Whilst this approach recognises the injuries done to the oppressed, they discounted the human psychodynamics and the sort of work that needed to be done beyond activism. Hence the need to put the radical into the relational and the relational into the radical.

The language used by the radical psychiatry group reflected the political mood of the time. The fighting spirit, the cry to battle, and the protesting voice was compelling in helping people unite and in gathering momentum for movements. That kind of voice is still heard again at times of political protest, and in recent times we have seen such passion with examples such as Black Lives Matter, Greta Thunberg, and climate change activists. As I write this, the Russian invasion of Ukraine is three months in progress with all the suffering, trauma, and terrible consequences that accompany such fighting. In the UK, it has given rise to protesting voices that have united across political party lines. This is not to discount the incidents of terrible racism that was/are being practised—especially on the borders. In contrast, the stories of refugees and asylum seekers from Afghanistan, Syria, and Africa have dissipated, as the government faces legal battles as to whether or not some of these people are forced to take a one-way flight to Rwanda. Historical experiences of war, of totalitarian states, and of forceful oppression have been ignited by what we are witnessing in the UK and other countries too, as people seem to be expressing their objections. The passion of these protests and the way these communications reach the world has developed since radio and camera. Social media is fast, can make an intense impact, and bypass the structures and processes of nationally approved communication channels, meaning it can be open to all and is currently without robust legislation. This has its advantages as well as concerns. Freedom of speech without ethics, responsibility, morality, and integrity gives rise to the sorts of hateful attacks that happen on social media presently, even with some safeguards in place. Much as we can hear so much more because of technical developments, and see news and evidence that might otherwise stay underground, social media has also facilitated our capacity to be reactive, impulsive, and at times vicious.

The complexity of our global networks and international dependencies gives rise during times of social and economic crisis to nationalistic turmoil that is infectious, influencing us all in a number of ways. Yet, the protective atmosphere and privacy of the consulting room can give the illusion of safety, meaning it may be a challenge to look outside that door and incorporate the realities of oppression, trauma, prejudice, entitlement, and other psychodynamics around privilege into clinical work. Whilst there may be a place for pride in one's country, a loyalty to the land we feel we belong to, nationalistic mindsets are at risk of totalitarian states of mind that erupt during times of war. War exposes the violence that is inherent in these states of mind, which Freud, Berne, and Bion thought about and wrote about. The impact of the World Wars and the rise of the Nazis influenced their thinking and their work. Social realities driven by the psychodynamics of economics penetrate our lives and our minds and therefore are relevant in clinical work.

Pressure groups exert important influence from outside the power base by challenging the reputation of those in power. Calling out social injustice continues to be important. However, there also needs to be bridge-building, especially with potential allies. The differences that can arise between and amongst oppressed groups is not helpful when they turn their battles on each other. There needs to be space for dialogue, broadening and deepening understanding in order to keep learning and strengthening. I have referred to this sort of dialogue as Anton Hart's "radical openness" (Hart, 2017). The calling out of our unconscious defences helps us see how we have internalised normative processes and normative language and unwittingly colluded with the power base. To see this helps us expand consciousness and make informed choices. The relational helps cross radical bridges and helps the dialogue so that people and potential allies do not become alienated from each other.

Recognising that systemic power once gained is hard to change from within, something of the "other" seems necessary. In Chapter Six, I wrote about Fiona Williams' referencing structures of feeling (F. Williams, 2021), which was a sociological reminder that communities develop their feelings about subjects in life and these pressure groups are therefore able to exert political influence based on these feelings. This has an impact on the power base, despite resistance within. As stated, those in power are usually keen to hold on to their frame of reference and their position. The pressure groups on the outside may raise awareness of deception (e.g., Thunberg challenging world leaders that COP26 was full of loopholes and was a PR exercise [BBC News, 2021]), which is helpful in pushing for a dialogue that might not otherwise happen. The capacity to have tenacity and single-mindedness is a show of determination, resilience, and courage in many circumstances. I am not pointing to the kind of single-mindedness that is related to defensiveness, rigidity, or splitting. Rather, I mean the kind of resilience and strength that is hard won. The kind that comes from knowing suffering, facing the challenge that experience evokes, and reaching a position that holds integrity for who we are. So, a protesting voice, a loud "NO", is to draw important lines for self, others, and communities.

In the radical reformation "formula", I proposed plurality as a goal—the capacity to move between positions, to know when we are up against our own internal oppressive processes, and we need to do battle within. In light of pluralism, how then can single-mindedness have a place? Do our philosophical and political positions, our weddedness to a particular approach with theory or social life mean we are all at risk of pushing our own states of mind, our own thoughts, and closing down on the other? At the other polarity, if we are constantly open and flexible does that risk us having no backbone at all? Of having no moral, ethical philosophical position—as if all perspectives are of equal value and merit? As Dalal (2012) writes:

> What I am against is an indiscriminate respect and tolerance that requires the tolerator to disengage from their own discriminatory processes. In doing so, they would be abandoning their own humanity as they suspended living according to the claims of their own ethics.
>
> (p. 246)

Dalal challenges the notion of therapeutic or social neutrality, calls upon us to hold a position, know what we stand for, and be clear of our values and be informed by them. I have argued that we need to be mindful of power dynamics and aware of the tendency of power to gravitate to the powerful and be held there. However, the path to recovery for the patient/client, however we might think of it, does not lie merely in shouting at authority figures, the establishment, or even the internal Parent ego state as we name it in Transactional Analysis. Rather, from a relational perspective, there is a requirement to retain our critical minds, create relatedness, dialogue, reflectiveness, regulation, and mentalisation.

In the opening chapter to this book, I considered the challenge within Transactional Analysis of having psychoanalytical roots yet developing practitioners along the way who leaned towards a behavioural and humanistic practice. The desire to believe in innate human goodness has allowed the discipline to develop and progress a capacity for compassion, support, and love. This has helped create bonds and affiliations—a network of communities that can come together and enjoy each other. However, there has been a loss too. The loss has been the felt experience behind our theories, a missing out of the depth and breadth of perspectives, and therefore it has not always been possible to have resilience in our relatedness with each other. Through a hunger and longing for safety, recognition, and love, our community has at times struggled to acknowledge and work with the shadow. The collective "Bad Me" is marginalised and evokers can end up as provokers who then get ostracised. This is possibly a reflection of the wider societies we live in. In this book I have argued that relational approaches have attempted to counteract this. They have encouraged depth. Then, a revisiting of the radical creates opportunity to open our eyes to power dynamics so that the corrupt, the envious, and the competitive can be seen, understood, and responded to.

These processes are challenging to address and require us to push ourselves to hold a strong-minded position alongside flexibility. These dynamics together can seem counter-intuitive. They could suggest a moderation of passion, a dissolving of clarity and position, and so I hope the reader has seen enough in this book to know that is not what I am suggesting. Rather, I am saying that when the going is tough, the capacity to hold on to our minds whilst moving between internal subjective states to relatedness, influence, and affectedness with others is ongoing work. The patient is not merely an innocent victim to an oppressive system but an active subject who has struggled with experiences of alienation alongside growing insight and wisdom. I believe the same is true for our experience of ourselves within our communities.

From Sickness Versus Health to Expanding Consciousness

The radical psychiatry movement opened up important dialogue about the impact of culture and systemic power dynamics on our minds. This had long been discounted in most models of psychotherapy, particularly in the West as we moved more and more into industrialisation, capitalism, and living in large urban spaces, the architecture of which drastically affected community feelings and spirit. We have been deceived into thinking the individual is a person that makes free choices as if they are not in any way influenced by their history and cultural frames of reference. Considering we need to work hard with our own internal states, be open-minded and flexible—yet also know what we stand for and what we fight for, I think it important to think about.

In Chapter Three I acknowledged Novellino's contribution to rules of communication in that he highlights the challenge of the therapist understanding and formulating the unconscious into words: words that can be used and responded to. I mentioned that neither Berne nor Novellino

150

tackled the experience of the therapist in coming to "know" what to say. The potential struggle within the therapist between their self-interest and their willingness to find a new perspective, a new way of experiencing and seeing their client is what makes the relational way of working radical. Transactional Analysis has developed over the years from a binary perspective of what is "healthy" or "unhealthy", to a more explorative sense of "what is it that needs to be understood here, and how are we going to expand and deepen our experiences of each other?" Radically speaking, analysing psychological transactions had originally developed into game analysis and a way of "correcting" the dishonesty of the deception. However, in the past, this often led to a sense of shaming the client and reinforcing a sense of "Bad Me" as I described in the game/enactment or re-enactment with my therapist in Chapter Eight. Shadbolt's extended game formula (Chapter Seven) illustrates the way in which our theories are to be launch pads for further thoughts and further development, and my proposal of radical reformation is in agreement with this.

The plurality that I was aiming to describe in my reformation formula includes the therapist's willingness to challenge themselves and stretch their own frame of reference, their perspective on the client, and the transferential situation, whilst still holding on to their own mind. As I have shown in my case examples, this can be difficult, even seemingly impossible at times, if the therapist is inclined to dissociate. Hence, the therapist's vulnerabilities are bound to come into play, especially when there is something critical and unconscious that is struggling to make itself known. Transactional Analysis has a bounty of clarifying models. It is in part what drew me to the discipline—the hope to make sense of my confusion. It is a very attractive feature of this paradigm. However, when the practitioner is feeling under-resourced, it may become too easy to rely on well-known ideas and concepts from the theories and overuse them to "diagnose" the difficulties of the patient/client. This can provide a sense of safety and stability for the practitioner in a situation that may feel unpredictable and unknown. Relying on theory in these circumstances can lead to an oppressive dynamic, which leaves the therapist comfortable, but missing the client and possibly projecting their own unprocessed material on to their client. The practitioner's role affords protection by being the one who could take the position of having answers and influencing the client to adapt to their mind and their needs. Chapter Four described this kind of complementary transaction and the psychological dynamics therein. Hence, anti-oppressive practice has to include a capacity in the therapist to be aware of their own defensiveness, their own vulnerabilities, and their own self-interest. I emphasise this as I think this is where professional and personal growth meet the ethics of radical Transactional Analysis. When defences are activated and pressure is put on therapeutic relating, I expect that a process of mutual change and growth is not happening, and something needs to get evoked to bring new vitality to the work. I have attempted to illustrate this in my case examples, such as those of Alan in Chapters Three and Seven, Emma in Chapters Four and Eight, and Colleen in Chapter Eight.

Reflections on Writing This Book

Given the importance of growth and change within the practitioner, I would like to comment on the ways in which I have been changed by writing this book. I could not have known what would emerge for me personally, however, as I progressed, many things were changed. The pace and timings were frequently revised. Unexpected world, national, and regional events made an impact and left a mark on me and provoked further thoughts and reflections on the themes I wanted to raise in this book. Looking back at the chapters, I have written about the dynamics of alienation, the process of mutual change, and possible social and personal liberation. I have shared the way the current contextual challenges affect me along with other citizens and professionals in the socio-political and psychological arenas. As a relational psychotherapist, I reiterate the case that in depth studies on mother/infant dyads have been tremendously helpful in understanding the development of emotional literacy, affect regulation, the capacity for intimacy, and making meaningful attachments and bonds. However, as a radical thinker, the overemphasis on the individual in Eurocentric philosophy is not enough. It does not account sufficiently for context and the power dynamics in personal and professional relationships. Taking account of how systemic dynamics impact on people and society continues to be critical to me and strengthens my belief that in order to move psychotherapy forward, it must not be left as an alienated discipline but seen as a valuable and critical part of contributing to healthy people, societies, and states. I think this is why there needs to be a greater emphasis on our ancestral and contemporary social and political contexts.

I started writing this book in 2018, expecting it to be a two-year project. A house and work move, family bereavement, responsibilities for care, and my personal transition from a difficult decade of peri-menopause to menopause meant that my expectations had to change. I am not one to miss a self-inflicted deadline, so extending the time, slowing and expanding the space between my endeavours, and lightening my workload in the process was a challenging personal adjustment. I literally had to find a new rhythm and a new mindset. What I needed to change on the inside also says something about the change in my external environment. I was settling into a new geography and a new landscape with new people around me. Internally and externally, it has been a radical and relational encounter.

I am a person who feels connected to three continents and who has lived in many places. It sometimes feels like I have wide rather than deep roots, and I have envied those who feel that deep connection to their place of birth, their land, and their landscapes, whether they be urban or rural. However, the movement of my predecessors, my people, and in my lifetime, myself, has brought me some benefits. It has demanded that I take in my surroundings, that I push myself to make a home where I settle, and that I open my mind and heart to the people that live around me—even though they may think and live differently from me. Having spent nearly two decades in one place, in a place which truly became a home, where I did garden and I did grow my own vegetables, moving again later in life did enlighten me that I had finally made a home in my adult life. It proved to be a deep wrench to leave it. There is much to enjoy in my current landscape, and it was important for me to come to this part of the UK. As I grow older, I wanted to feel connected to the land and to the seasons and there is enormous scope to do that in the south-west of England. It is also a reflection of the privilege I have gained in my adult life in that I have choices about where I can go. This freedom of movement is a radical thing and a huge privilege. Much as my race is more visible here than in many other parts of the UK, I can wear my skin with more ease, and having some modest material comfort also makes life comfortable in many respects.

As the time I was taking to complete was stretched, I had limited capacity to immerse and focus. My fear grew that my writing would all be too late, that I would miss the mood of the time and, as I saw it, the necessity for more political writing. As I have described, writing about my radical and relational approach has been motivated by the impact of what has been happening in my country and the rest of the world through my middle years. However, the other texts that have been written and published through this era of my life help me realise that I am not alone. I am grateful for this. In the past few years, new and innovative political writing has come into the psychological fields and has shown how the political is the professional and the personal. These authors and practitioners have felt very much like allies, and I have referenced many of them in this book. I would like to highlight a few that like me, have focused on the political and the psychological. I am grateful for the inspiration from Wieland (2015) and Keval (2016), the directness of Turner (2021), the compassion of Ellis (2021), and the creativity of Foluke Taylor. Recently, I have also been glad to meet Valerie Sinason and learn from her insight, compassion, and experience of working with war trauma and refugees. On November 28, 2020, Robert Downes and Foluke Taylor led a conference online (the International Association of Relational Transactional Analysis [IARTA]), and one of the suggestions from Taylor was to create a playlist for a course you are designing or the book you are writing. I loved this refreshing idea and made an extensive list of songs and music that have inspired me personally, politically, and emotionally. I won't list them all here, but have restricted myself to one per chapter. To conclude the book, I share some of the music and songs that have been inspirational and meant something to me. In the spirit of the times, I offer a link to YouTube for each.

Thank you for reading—it means a lot to write, and even more to be read.

Playlist

Chapter One

The Sound of Silence—Simon & Garfunkel https://www.youtube.com/watch?v=NAEppFUWLfc

Chapter Two

One in Ten—UB40 https://www.youtube.com/watch?v=quTIjiw1xGE

Chapter Three

Under Pressure—David Bowie and Queen https://www.youtube.com/watch?v=DZBCUfGAbN8

Chapter Four

I've Been Dead 400 Years—Jimmy Cliff https://www.youtube.com/watch?v=gMmqcZmKk4U

Chapter Five

Redemption Song—Bob Marley https://www.youtube.com/watch?v=Md8EesTaIsA
Do Dilon Ke—Shreya Ghoshal, Hariharan, and A.R. Rahman https://www.youtube.com/watch?v=A-Y7ehp9qL0

Chapter Six

Free Nelson Mandela—Special AKA https://www.youtube.com/watch?v=rLMV7Buj5g0

Chapter Seven

I Want to Break Free—Queen https://www.youtube.com/watch?v=f4Mc-NYPHaQ

Chapter Eight

I Am I Said—Neil Diamond https://www.youtube.com/watch?v=7p330-ecXvs

Chapter Nine

Kurigalu Saar kurigalu—MD pallavi | GKVK Kannada tingala habba https://www.youtube.com/watch?v=5gYDp8PerSc

Chapter Eleven

Many Rivers to Cross—Jimmy Cliff https://www.youtube.com/watch?v=kGeCeK85sUg

Note

1 My thanks to Keith Tudor (personal communication, November 12, 2018) for offering this exploration.

GLOSSARY OF TECHNICAL TERMS

Alienation A term originally used by Karl Marx to describe the loss of meaning to work and relationships.

Alienation formula Oppression + Deception = Alienation, Attributed to Hogie Wycoff. She wrote that alienation as a process requires a dynamic of oppression along with deceiving the oppressed.

"Bad Me" A state of mind resisted yet identified with by an individual that undermines their self-esteem. Usually it evokes feelings of shame.

Collective A state of mind shared by the majority.

Counterscript A system of being for the individual that is an adaptation to social norms, helps them to function and keep deeper defences at bay.

Countertransference Conscious and unconscious responses to communication from another.

Decontamination A process through which defensive and limiting unconscious beliefs come into awareness.

Dissociative processes Dynamics whereby people disconnect completely from thinking, feeling, memories, awareness and/or identity.

Drivers Pre-conscious processes used to adapt to an authority figure or system. They are usually accompanied by mild to moderate feelings of anxiety and they defend against deeper feelings of inadequacy.

Ego states Distinct systems in the mind for feelings, beliefs, reactions and responses.

Empathic Specification A therapeutic intervention to articulate the felt understanding from specification the therapist of the underlying theme or significance within the client's communication.

Empathic Transactions A range of therapeutic interventions that convey empathy to the Transactions client.

Enactment Unconscious behaviour erupting from a dissociative state of mind.

Extractive Introjection A term defined by Christopher Bollas to describe the process of robbing another of their psychological resources.

Games Repetitive defensive manoeuvres between people that lead to limiting or destructive outcomes.

Injunctions Unconscious self limiting or destructive inhibiting messages usually delivered by carers and taken on by the individual during childhood.

Intersectionality A term originally defined by Crenshaw to describe the interactions of different social identities, some of which evoke experiences of oppression in society.

Introjection A process of consciously or unconsciously internalising aspects of another's state of mind.

"Not Me" A state of mind or an identity that feels alien to the individual.

Physis The vital and spiritual force for life.

Projective Identification A state of feeling, usually disturbing that has been unconsciously communicated from one person to another. The recipient can only experience it if they identify with it.

Racket feelings Defensive feelings that are usually more accepting to experience than the congruent one.

Reclamation A term used in this book to recover lost states of mind.

Redecisional A way of treating internal conflicts via activating regression to re-experience the historical injury and change the outcome.

Re-Enactment A term used in this book to describe a re-experiencing of a historical trauma.

Resurrection A term used in this book to describe the return of psychological vitality after long periods of dissociation.

Ruptures Experiences that break trust or the therapeutic alliance.

Script A defensive psychological system that is self-limiting or destructive for the individual. It is unconscious and is created from life or relational stress.

Script decisions Unconscious self-limiting decisions that help the individual survive a social and/or psychological system.

Script protocol Early relational failures in an infant's experience that lay down their emotional blueprint.

Social adaptations These are adaptations to society and may include both counterscript and script.

Spontaneous Consent A term used to describe automatic surrender to the demands or oppression from a more powerful other.

Symbiosis Dependencies on a system or authority figure that is activated and desired by the powerful.

Transactions Communications between people.

Transference drama Unconscious communications between people that repeat relational dynamics from the past.

Transferential relationship A therapeutic relationship between client and therapist that seeks to understand past relational dynamics by making use of the subjective experiences in both parties.

Transferential Transaction An unconscious communication usually used to mean from the client that includes their experience of the therapist based on past relational dynamics.

Winner A term used by Eric Berne to describe a person whose adaptation to society offers them rewards.

Winning formulas A strategy, usually defensive that nonetheless offers rewards.

Winning Scripts A term used by Eric Berne to denote unconscious life plans that are defensive yet offer rewards to the individuals.

REFERENCES

Achebe, C. (1958). *Things fall apart*. Heinemann Educational Books.

Angelou, M. (1986). *And still I rise*. Virago Press.

Batts, V. (1982). Modern racism: A TA perspective. *Transactional Analysis Journal, 12*(3), 207–209. 10.1177/036215378201200309.

BBC News. (2017, August 1). *Cyril Radcliffe: The man who drew the partition line*. https://www.bbc.com/news/av/world-asia-40788079.

BBC News. (2021, November 15). *Greta Thunberg says 'many loopholes' in COP26 pact*. https://www.bbc.com/news/uk-scotland-glasgow-west-59296859.

BBC Sport. (2021, November 6). *Yorkshire County Cricket Club investigating after another ex-player alleges racial abuse*. https://www.bbc.com/sport/cricket/59186071.

Benjamin, J. (1988). *Bonds of love*. Pantheon Books.

Berges, P. M., Chadha, G., & Nayar, D. (Producers). (2017). *Viceroy's House* [Film]. 20th Century Fox.

Berne, E. (1947). *The mind in action*. Simon & Schuster.

Berne, E. (1961). *Transactional analysis in psychotherapy: A systematic individual and social psychiatry*. Grove Press. 10.1037/11495-000.

Berne, E. (1963). *Structure and dynamics of groups and organisations*. Ballantine Books.

Berne, E. (1964). *Games people play: The psychology of human relationships*. Grove Press.

Berne, E. (1972). *What do you say after you say hello?* Grove Press.

Berne, E. (1975). *What do you say after you say hello?* Corgi.

Berne, E. (2020). Man as a political animal. *Psychotherapy and Politics International, 18*(3), e1568. 10.1002/ppi.1568.

Biko, S. (1978). *I write what I like*. Heinemann.

Bion, W. R. (1959). Attacks on linking. *The International Journal of Psychoanalysis, 40*, 308–315.

Bion, W. R. (2010). *Experiences in groups*. Routledge. (Original work published 1961).

Blackstone, P. (1993). The dynamic child: Integration of second-order structure, object relations, and self psychology. *Transactional Analysis Journal, 23*(4), 216–234. 10.1177/036215379302300406.

Bollas, C. (1987). *The shadow of the object: Psychoanalysis of the unthought known*. Free Association Books.

Bowater, M. (2003). Windows on your inner self: Dreamwork with transactional analysis. *Transactional Analysis Journal, 33(1)*, 37–44. 10.1177/0362153703033 00106.

Burley, L. (Director). (2017a, August 9). *My family, partition and me: India 1947, Episode one* [TV series episode]. British Broadcasting Corporation.

Burley, L. (Director). (2017b, August 16). *My family, partition and me: India 1947, Episode two* [Television programme]. British Broadcasting Corporation.

Butler, P. (2021, January 21). Rashford demands a 'meal a day' for all school pupils in need. *The Guardian*. https://www.theguardian.com/education/2021/jan/20/rashford-demands-a-meal-a-day-for-all-school-pupils-in-need.

Chinnock, K., & Minikin, K. (2015). Multiple contemporaneous games in psychotherapy: Psychodynamic and political perspectives. *Transactional Analysis Journal, 45(2)*, 141–152. 10.1177/0362153715585096.

Clark, B. (1991). Empathic transactions in the deconfusion of the child ego states. *Transactional Analysis Journal, 21(2)*, 92–98. 10.1177/036215379102100204.

Clarkson, P. (1993). Transactional analysis as a humanistic therapy. *Transactional Analysis Journal, 23(1)*, 36–41. 10.1177/036215379302300104.

Cornell, W. F. (2018). If it is not for all, it is not for us: Reflections on racism, nationalism, and populism in the United States. *Transactional Analysis Journal, 48(2)*, 97–110. 10.1080/03621537.2018.1431460.

Cornell, W. F. (2020). Transactional analysis and psychoanalysis: Overcoming the narcissism of small differences in the shadow of Eric Berne. *Transactional Analysis Journal, 50(3)*, 164–178. 10.1080/03621537.2020.1771020.

Cornell, W. F., & Bonds-White, F. (2001). Therapeutic relatedness in transactional analysis: The truth of love or the love of truth. *Transactional Analysis Journal, 31(1)*, 71–83. 10.1177/036215370103100108.

Cornell, W. F., & Landaiche, N. M. (2006). Impasse and intimacy: Applying Berne's concept of script protocol. *Transactional Analysis Journal, 36(3)*, 196–213. 10.1177/036215370603600304.

Cowburn, A. (2020, February 14). Boris Johnson cabinet now two-thirds privately educated after reshuffle, compared to 7% of UK population. *The Independent*. https://www.independent.co.uk/news/uk/politics/boris-johnson-cabinet-reshuffle-news-privately-educated-mps-a9335261.html.

Crenshaw, K. (1989). *Demarginalizing the intersection of race and sex: A black feminist criique of antidiscrimination doctrine, feminist theory and antiracist politics*. https://chicagounbound.uchicago.edu/cgi/viewcontent.cgi?article=1052&context=uclf.

Dalal, F. (2012). *Thought paralysis: The virtues of discrimination*. Karnac Books.

Dalal, F. (2018). *CBT: The cognitive behavioural tsunami*. Routledge.

Derrida, J. (1967). *Writing and difference*. Éditions du Seuil.

DeYoung, P. A. (2003). *Relational psychotherapy: A primer*. Routledge. 10.4324/9781315810911.

Dhananjaya, D. (2022). We are the oppressor and the oppressed: The interplay between intrapsychic, interpersonal, and societal intersectionality. *Transactional Analysis Journal, 52(3)*, 244–258. 10.1080/03621537.2022.2082031.

Diamond, N. (1971). I am ... I said [Song]. On *Hot August Night*. MCA.

Dirks, N. B. (1989). The original caste: Power, history and hierarchy in South Asia. *Contributions to Indian Sociology, 23(1)*, 59–77. 10.1177/006996689023001005.

Ellis, E. (2021). *The race conversation: An essential guide to creating life-changing dialogue*. Confer Books.

English, F. (1971). The substitution factor: Rackets and real feelings. *Transactional Analysis Journal, 1(4)*, 27–32. 10.1177/036215377100100408.

English, F. (1996). Berne, phobia, episcripts, and racketeering. *Transactional Analysis Journal, 26(2)*, 122–131. 10.1177/036215379602600203.

Erskine, R. (1993). Inquiry, attunement, and involvement in the psychotherapy of dissociation. *Transactional Analysis Journal, 23(4)*, 184–190. 10.1177/0362153793 02300402.

Erskine, R., & Zalcman, M. (1979). The racket system: A model for racket analysis. *Transactional Analysis Journal, 9(1)*, 51–59. 10.1177/036215377900900112.

Fanon, F. (2021). *Black skin, white masks*. Penguin Modern Classics. (Original work published 1952)

Fisher, M. (2009). *Capitalist realism: Is there no alternative?* John Hunt Publishing Ltd.

Fonagy, P., Gergely, G., Jurist, E., & Target, M. (2002). *Affect regulation, mentalization and the development of self*. Taylor and Francis Ltd.

Fromm, E. (1956). *The sane society*. Routledge.

Fromm, E. (2009). *Beyond the chains of illusion*. Continuum. (Original work published 1962)

Gallagher, M., Smith, T., & Adeane, A. (Producers). (2017a, August 7). *Partition voices: Aftermath. Episode one* [Radio programme]. British Broadcasting Corporation. https://www.bbc.co.uk/programmes/b09013nl.

Gallagher, M., Smith, T., & Adeane, A. (Producers). (2017b, August 14). *Partition voices: Division. Episode two* [Radio programme]. British Broadcasting Corporation. https://www.bbc.co.uk/programmes/b08z9p9w.

Gallagher, M., Smith, T., & Adeane, A. (Producers). (2017c, August 21). *Partition voices: Legacy. Episode three* [Radio programme]. British Broadcasting Corporation. https://www.bbc.co.uk/programmes/b090wg29.

Gerhardt, S. (2004). *Why love matters: How affection shapes a baby's brain*. Routledge.

Gramsci, A. (2003). *Selections from prison notebooks*. Lawrence and Wishart. (Original work published 1971)

Hall, S. (2017). *Familiar stranger: A life between two islands* (B. Schwarz, Ed.). Penguin.

Hanisch, C. (1969). *The personal is political*. http://www.carolhanisch.org/CHwritings/PIP.html.

Hargaden, H., & Sills, C. (2001). Deconfusion of the child ego state: A relational perspective. *Transactional Analysis Journal, 31(1)*, 55–70. 10.1177/036215370103100107.

Hargaden, H., & Sills, C. (2002). *Transactional analysis: A relational perspective*. Brunner-Routledge.

Harris, T. (1967). *I'm OK, you're OK*. Harper and Row.

Hart, A. (2017). From multicultural competence to radical openness: A psychoanalytic engagement of otherness. *The American Psychoanalyst, 51(1)*. https://apsa.org/apsaa-publications/vol51no1-TOC/html/vol51no1_09.xhtml.

Hart, A. (2022). from multicultural competence to radical openness: A psychoanalytic engagement of otherness. In B. J. Stoute & M. Slevin (Eds.), *The trauma of racism* (pp. 244–250). Routledge.

REFERENCES

Holding, M. (2021). *Why we kneel, how we rise*. Simon and Schuster.

Hussain, A. (1966). *Pakistan: Its ideology and foreign policy*. Frank Cass and Co. Ltd.

Johnson, S. (2017). The trouble with gender. *Transactional Analysis Journal, 47(4)*, 308–320. 10.1177/0362153717725533.

Keval, N. (2016). *Racist states of mind: Understanding the perversion of curiosity and concern*. Karnac Books.

Kriegman, D., & Slavin, M. (1998). Why the analyst needs to change: Toward a theory of conflict, negotiation and mutual influence in the therapeutic process. *Psychoanalytic Dialogues, 8(2)*, 247–284. 10.1080/10481889809539246.

Layard, R. (2005). *Happiness*. Penguin.

Layton, L. (2020). *Toward a social psychoanalysis: Culture, character, and normative unconscious processes*. Routledge.

Lewis, P. (2019, June 22). Exploring the rise of populism: 'It pops up in unexpected places'. *The Guardian*. https://www.theguardian.com/membership/2019/jun/22/populism-new-exploring-rise-paul-lewis.

Little, R. (2006). Ego state relational units and resistance to change. *Transactional Analysis Journal, 36(1)*, 7–9. 10.1177/036215370603600103.

Little, R. (2013). The new emerges out of the old. *Transactional Analysis Journal, 43(2)*, 106–121. 10.1177/0362153713499541.

Luther King, M. (1963). *From a gift of love: Sermons from strength to love*. Penguin Modern Classics.

Lynch, W. (1712). *The Making of a Slave*.

Marley, B. (1980). Redemption Song [Song]. On *Uprising*. Island Records.

Marx. (1967). The process of production of capital. In F. Engels (Ed.) and S. Moore & E. Aveling (Trans), *Capital: A critique of political economy* (Vol. *1*). Progress Publishers.

Maslow, A. (1943). A theory of human motivation. *Psychological Review, 50(4)*, 370–396.

Mellor, K. (1980). Impasses: A developmental and structural understanding. *Transactional Analysis Journal, 10(3)*, 213–220. 10.1177/036215378001000307.

MHFA England. (2020). *Mental health statistics*. https://mhfaengland.org/mhfa-centre/research-and-evaluation/mental-health-statistics/.

Miller, E. (1998). Are basic assumptions instinctive? In F. Borgogno, S. A. Merciai, & P. Bion Talamo (Eds.), *Bion's Legacy to Groups*. Routledge.

Minikin, K. (2011). Transactional analysis and the wider world: The politics and psychology of alienation. In H. Fowlie & C. Sills (Eds.), *Relational transactional analysis: Principles in practice*. Karnac Books.

Minikin, K. (2018). Radical relational psychiatry: Toward a democracy of mind and people. *Transactional Analysis Journal, 48(2)*, 111–125. 10.1080/03621537.2018.1429287.

Minikin, K. (2020). Transactional analysis and our philosophical premises: 70 years on. *Psychotherapy and Politics International, 18(3)*. 10.1002/ppi.1563.

Minikin, K. (2021). Relative privilege and the seduction of normativity. *Transactional Analysis Journal*, 1–12. 10.1080/03621537.2020.1853349.

Minikin, K., & Tudor, K. (2015). Gender psychopolitics: Men becoming, being and belonging. In R. Erskine (Ed.), *Transactional analysis in contemporary psychotherapy* (pp. 257–275). Karnac Books.

Minority Rights Group International. (2008). *World Directory of Minorities and Indigenous Peoples—India: Dalits.* https://www.refworld.org/docid/49749d13c.html.

Moiso, C. (1985). Ego states and transference. *Transactional Analysis Journal, 15(3),* 194–201. 10.1177/036215378501500302.

Morgan-Jones, R. (2010). *The body of the organisation and its health.* Karnac Books.

Morrison, T. (1988). *Beloved.* Pan Books.

NHS. (2019). *NHS mental health implementation plan 2019/20–2023/24.* https://www.longtermplan.nhs.uk/wp-content/uploads/2019/07/nhs-mental-health-implementation-plan-2019-20-2023-24.pdf.

Nissar Ahmed, K. S. (2003, January). Kurigalu, Saar, kurigalu [Poem]. In *Nityotsava (A Collection of Kannada Lyrics)* (9th ed., p. 39). Sapna Book House.

Noriega, G. (2010). The transgenerational script of transactional analysis. *Transactional Analysis Journal, 40(3–4),* 196–204. 10.1177/036215371004000304.

Novak, E. T. (2015). Are games, enactments, and reenactments similar? No, yes, it depends. *Transactional Analysis Journal, 45,* 117–127. 10.1177/0362153715578840.

Novak, E. T. (2022). emancipation from a fear of institutionalization: A case study of transgenerational hauntings. *Transactional Analysis Journal, 52(2),* 106–119. 10.1080/03621537.2022.2044112.

Novellino, M. (2005). Transactional psychoanalysis: Epistemological foundations. *Transactional Analysis Journal, 35(2),* 157–172. 10.1177/036215370503500206.

Ogden, T. H. (1979). On projective identification. *The International Journal of Psychoanalysis, 60(3),* 357–373.

Orbach, S. (2019, August 23). Will this be the last generation to have bodies that are familiar to us? *The Guardian.* https://www.theguardian.com/books/2019/aug/23/susie-orbach-that-will-bodies-be-like-in-the-future.

Quah, N., & Davis, L. E. (2015, May 2). *Here's a timeline of unarmed Black people killed by police over past year.* BuzzFeedNews. https://www.buzzfeednews.com/article/nicholasquah/heres-a-timeline-of-unarmed-black-men-killed-by-police-over.

Riley, S. (Director). (2010). *Fire in Babylon* [Documentary]. Cowboy Films; Passion Pictures.

Rogers, C. R. (1959). A theory of therapy, personality, and interpersonal relationships as developed in the client-centered framework. In S. Koch (Ed.), *Psychology: A study of a science* (Vol. 3, pp. 184–256). McGraw-Hill.

Savage, M. (2021, January 3). Richest 1% have almost a quarter of UK wealth, study claims. *The Guardian.* https://www.theguardian.com/inequality/2021/jan/03/richest-1-have-almost-a-quarter-of-uk-wealth-study-claims.

Schiff, A. W., & Lee Schiff, J. (1971). Passivity. *Transactional Analysis Bulletin, 1(1),* 71–78. 10.1177/036215377100100114.

Searles, H. F. (1955). The informational value of the supervisor's emotional experiences. *Psychiatry: Journal for the Study of Interpersonal Processes, 18,* 135–146.

Sedgwick, J. (2021). *Contextual transactional analysis: the inseparability of self and world.* Routledge.

Seelye, K. Q. (2020, July 17). John Lewis, towering figure of civil rights era, dies at 80. *The New York Times.* https://www.nytimes.com/2020/07/17/us/john-lewis-dead.html.

Shadbolt, C. (2012). The place of failure and rupture in psychotherapy. *Transactional Analysis Journal, 42(1),* 5–16. 10.1177/036215371204200102.

REFERENCES

Shaw, D. (2014). *Traumatic narcissism: Relational systems of subjugation.* Routledge.

Singh, N. I. (2002). *Communal violence in the Punjab 1947* [Unpublished doctoral dissertation]. Guru Nanak Dev University.

Stark, M. (1999). *Modes of therapeutic action.* Jason Aronson.

Steiner, C. (1997). *Achieving emotional literacy.* Bloomsbury.

Steiner, C. (2008). Eric Berne's politics: "The great pyramid". *Transactional Analysis Journal, 40(3–4)*, 212–216. 10.1177/036215371004000306.

Steiner, C., Wyckoff, H., Marcus, J., Lariviere, P., Goldstine, D., Schwebel, R., & Members of the Radical Psychiatry Center. (1975). *Readings in radical psychiatry.* Grove Press.

Stern, D. B. (2011). *Partners in thought: Working with unformulated experience, dissociation, and enactment.* Routledge.

Stuthridge, J. (2006). Inside out: A transactional analysis model of trauma. *Transactional Analysis Journal, 36(4)*, 270–283. 10.1177/036215370603600403.

Stuthridge, J. (2012). Traversing the fault lines: Trauma and enactment. *Transactional Analysis Journal, 42(4)*, 238–251. 10.1177/036215371204200402.

Stuthridge, J. (2015). All the world's a stage: Games, enactment, and counter-transference. *Transactional Analysis Journal, 45(2)*, 104–116. 10.1177/03621537155 81174.

Stuthridge, J. (2017). Falling apart and getting it together: The dialectics of dis-integration and integration in script change and self-development. *Transactional Analysis Journal, 47(1)*, 19–31. 10.1177/0362153716681029.

Sullivan, H. S. (1953). *The interpersonal theory of psychiatry.* W.W. Norton & Company.

Summers, G., & Tudor, K. (2000). Cocreative transactional analysis. *Transactional Analysis Journal, 30(1)*, 23–40. 10.1177/036215370003000104.

Summers, G., & Tudor, K. (2015). *Cocreative transactional analysis.* Karnac Books.

TACS. (2006). *Institutionalized oppression definitions.* https://sdmiramar.edu/sites/default/files/documents/2020-08/Communication%20&%20Collaboration%20Presentation%20Resources%208-13-20.pdf.

Talbot, I., & Singh, G. (2009). *The partition of India.* Cambridge University Press.

Tudor, K. (2008). "Take It": A sixth driver. *Transactional Analysis Journal, 38(1)*, 43–57. 10.1177/036215370803800107.

Tudor, K. (2016). "We are". The fundamental life position. *Transactional Analysis Journal, 46(2)*, 164–176. 10.1177/0362153716637064.

Turner, D. (2021). *Intersections of privilege and otherness in counselling and psycho-therapy.* Routledge.

CSL_BIBLIOGRAPHY Lynch, W. (1712). *The Making of a Slave.*

Van der Kolk, B. (2015). *The body keeps the score: Mind, brain and body in the transformation of trauma.* Penguin.

Wieland, C. (2015). *The fascist state of mind and the manufacturing of masculinity.* Routledge.

Wikipedia. (2022). *Viceroy's House* [Film]. https://en.wikipedia.org/wiki/Viceroy%27s_House_(film).

Wikipedia. (2023). *Scramble for Africa.* https://en.wikipedia.org/wiki/Scramble_for_Africa.

Williams, F. (2021). *Social policy: A critical and intersectional analysis*. Polity Press.

Williams, R. (1977). *Marxism and literature*. Oxford University Press.

Winnicott, D. W. (1953). Transitional objects and transitional phenomena: A study of the first not-me possession. *The International Journal of Psychoanalysis, 34*, 89–97.

Winnicott, D. W. (1960). Ego distortion in terms of true and false self. In *The maturational process and the facilitating environment*. Studies in the theory of emotional development (pp. 140–157). International Universities Press.

Yeats, W. B. (1919). *The Second Coming*.

Yerkes, R. M., & Dodson, J. D. (1908). The relation of strength of stimulus to rapidity of habit-formation. *Journal of Comparative Neurology and Psychology, 18*(5), 459–482. 10.1002/cne.920180503.

INDEX

INDEX

psychoanalysis 83
psychological change 11
psychological distress 83
psychotherapist, role of 24–25
psychotherapy 3, 17
public broadcasting 84

racket feelings 8, 157
Radcliffe, Cyril 72
radical psychiatry 4, 14, 16, 81, 83–87, 139, 147, 150
radical reformation 36, 149, 151
Rainford-Brent, Ebony 37
Rashford, Marcus 37
reclamation 99, 101–103; *Alan* (case example) 104–106; awakening and disturbance 106–108; in original form 110–111; radical relational reformation 108–109; relational connection and awakening 109–110; scripting process 103–104; Shadbolt's extended game formula 111–112
redecision approach 86, 133, 157
re-enactment 101, 114–115, 151, 157
relational psychotherapy 12, 131, 142–143
relational trauma 3, 49, 115, 128–129
relative privilege 91–93
remote working 21
repressive defences 128
resurrection 100, 109, 113, 157
retributive genocide 71
rivalry 45
Rogers, C. R. 132
rules of communication 150
ruptures 8, 111, 144, 157
Russia 68, 147
Rwanda 68

script 101–102, 114; decisions 5, 157; as double agent 48–50; process of 103–104; protocol 3, 40, 157; protocol and enactments 40
Sedgwick, James 21, 24, 102, 104, 111
self-alienation 103
self-expressions 103
self-sacrifice 128
self-sufficiency 24
sense of self 51
Shadbolt, C. 32, 103–104, 111–112, 151
shadeism 61–62, 90
Shakespeare 117

shaming 36, 48, 111–112, 151
Shaw, D. 114
Sinason, Valerie 153
skills building 136
slavery 17, 44–45, 57–59; abolition of 69; and gender politics 126–127
Slavin, M. 99
sleep, and transgenerational trauma 123–126
social adaptations 13, 157
social constructivism 15
social identity 80
socialism 6
social liberation 83–84; belongings 91; *Dani* (case example) 96–98; personal illustration 90–91; radical psychiatry and path to 84–87; radical relational reformation 99–100; relational and radical 93–96; relative privilege 91–93; sociological and psychoanalytical context 87–90
social media 84, 148
social mobility 75
social neutrality 149
societal oppression 137
sociology, and psychoanalysis 88–89
socio-political therapists 140–142
soul healing 100
spontaneity 6, 133
spontaneous consent 52, 121, 157
Steiner, Claude 4–5, 9–10, 138; early days of transactional analysis 5–6; psychological freedom 84
Stern, D. B. 109
structures of feelings 88
Sullivan, H. S. 39, 104–106, 109
survival 128
symbiosis 43–44, 70, 114, 157
Syria 27–28, 46

Taylor, Foluke 153
"Teacher–Student" dynamics 137
television 84
Thanatos 117–118
therapeutic neutrality 149
therapy 140
Things Fall Apart (Achebe) 51
Thunberg, Greta 84, 147–148
Transactional Analysis (TA) 3, 5; Berne's 5–6; current 11–12; early days 5–6; "I'm OK/You're OK" 7–9; people can change 10–11; people can

169

For Product Safety Concerns and Information please contact our EU
representative GPSR@taylorandfrancis.com
Taylor & Francis Verlag GmbH, Kaufingerstraße 24, 80331 München, Germany